Cerebral Lateralization

Cerebral Lateralization

Biological Mechanisms,
Associations,
and Pathology

Norman Geschwind, M.D.
Albert M. Galaburda, M.D.

A Bradford Book
The MIT Press
Cambridge, Massachusetts
London, England

Much of this book appeared as a three-part article in the "Archives of Neurology," Volume 42, May, June, and July, 1985.

This book was set in Palatino by Achorn Graphic Services, Inc. and printed and bound by Halliday Lithograph in the United States of America.

Library of Congress Cataloging-in-Publication Data

Geschwind, Norman.
  Cerebral lateralization.

  "A Bradford book."
  Bibliography: p.
  Includes index.
  1. Brain—Localization of functions.   2. Cerebral
dominance.   3. Diseases—Causes and theories of
causation.   I. Galaburda, Albert M., 1948–   .
II. Title.   [DNLM: 1. Dominance, Cerebral.
WL 335 G389c]
QP385.G47   1987   612'.825   86-10373
ISBN 0-262-07101-0

To Patricia Dougan Geschwind

Contents

Acknowledgments

It will be evident in these pages how indebted we are to Peter Behan of the University of Glasgow and to Thomas Kemper. We would also like to express our gratitude to many other individuals whose work or personal comments have especially influenced our approach to different issues. Much of whatever may be useful is the direct outgrowth of their stimulation, but they are not responsible for any erroneous facts or conclusions. We apologize for any omissions in this list.

We are indebted to (in alphabetical order) B. A. Afzelius, Marian Annett, Charles Boklage, Patrick Bray, Michael Corballis, Martha Denckla, Victor Denenberg, Marian Diamond, Gunter Dorner, Jack Fishman, Pierre Flor-Henry, Stanley Glick, Patricia Goldman-Rakic, Roger Gorski, J. A. Gustafsson, Paul Ivanyi, Robert Lahita, Nicole LeDouarin, Jerre Levy, Christie Ludlow, Richard Masland, Michael Morgan, Charles Netley, Fernando Nottebohm, Christopher Ounsted, Philip Paterson, Geoffrey Raisman, Pasko Rakic, David Rosenfield, Arnold Scheibel, Richard Sidman, John Simpson, David C. Taylor, Juhn Wada, and the late Paul Yakovlev. Special thanks are due to our coworkers Francisco Aboitiz, Heiko Braak, William DeBassio, David Eidelberg, Olaf Heine, Marjorie LeMay, Deepak Pandya, Glenn Rosen, Marjorie Ross, Friedrich Sanides, Gordon Sherman, and Steven Schachter and to our colleagues of the Neurology Department of the Beth Israel Hospital and the Psychology Department of the Massachusetts Institute of Technology.

We express our warm thanks to Loraine Karol for her devotion to the preparation of the many drafts of this book, to Patricia Geschwind for preparing the bibliography, and to Anne Mark for her expert editing help.

The work reported here was supported in part by grants from the National Science Foundation, the National Institutes of Health, the Orton Research Fund, and the Essel Foundation.

1   Introduction

We present a set of hypotheses about the biological mechanisms of lateralization, the processes that lead to an asymmetrical nervous system. It would have been difficult even twenty years ago to formulate such a theory in the face of the prevalent belief that cerebral dominance lacked an anatomical correlate. It is proposed that cerebral dominance is based in most instances on asymmetries of structure. Although we know that genetic factors are important, we will emphasize several factors that modify the direction and extent of these structural differences in the course of development, both prenatal and postnatal. We will direct special attention to the intrauterine environment (and, in particular, sex hormones or related factors) as a determinant of the pattern of asymmetries. We will discuss the associations of anomalous cerebral dominance, which will include not only developmental disorders such as dyslexia and certain talents but also alterations in many bodily systems, including the immune system, the skin, and the skeleton. We propose that the same influences that modify structural asymmetry in the brain also modify other systems.

We begin in chapter 2 by reviewing briefly the history of some concepts of cerebral dominance, or functional asymmetry within the brain. In chapter 3 we summarize the essentials of our theory of lateralization, supporting this theory in subsequent chapters with detailed data on the biological mechanisms and associations of cerebral dominance. Among the studies reported in those chapters are certain major findings that have stimulated our studies and theoretical considerations. By way of both preview and overview, we summarize those studies here.

1. *Anatomical asymmetry of the brain.* It has been demonstrated (Geschwind and Levitsky 1968) and later confirmed in several studies

that the human brain exhibits an easily detectable asymmetry involving the upper surface of the posterior portion of the left temporal lobe. Because this region, the *planum temporale*, constitutes a large portion of the temporal speech region of Wernicke, asymmetry of this zone may account for the predominant localization of speech to the left hemisphere in the majority of humans. Other asymmetries in the human brain have been described (LeMay and Culebras 1972; Galaburda, et al. 1978). The larger size of the left planum temporale reflects the greater extent of a particular cytoarchitectonic area (Tpt) on the left (Galaburda, Sanides, and Geschwind 1978).

2. *Asymmetry of the fetal brain.* Asymmetry is found in the brain of the human fetus and newborn infant, thus establishing the importance of genetic and/or intrauterine influences (Wada, Clarke, and Hamm 1975; Witelson and Pallie 1973; Chi, Dooling, and Gilles 1977).

3. *Male-female differences in the brain.* A higher frequency of left-handedness among males has been reported in many studies (Oldfield 1971), although not in all. Recent studies support the view that males and females differ on the average in their patterns of abilities (Maccoby and Jacklin 1974; Wittig and Petersen 1979; Benbow and Stanley 1980). Males predominate among cases of autism, dyslexia, stuttering, and other developmental disorders (Taylor 1974).

4. *Laterality in developmental disorders.* Many studies have reported elevated rates of lefthandedness in autism, stuttering, dyslexia, and other developmental disorders, although other studies have failed to find this correlation (Hécaen 1984). We have found a markedly higher rate of dyslexia and stuttering among strong lefthanders than among strong righthanders (Geschwind and Behan 1982, 1984).

5. *Abnormal cytoarchitecture in childhood dyslexia.* The cortex of a severe childhood dyslexic studied in our laboratory contains an abnormal pattern of cytoarchitecture virtually confined to the left hemisphere, in particular the temporal speech region. These anomalies are the result of disordered neuronal migration and/or assembly (Galaburda and Kemper 1979). The brain of a second dyslexic patient has abnormalities of neuronal architecture in the same regions (Galaburda 1983; Kemper 1984), and we have evidence for similar anomalies in living patients with arteriovenous malformations in the left temporal region. Postmortem brains of two other dyslexics have similar anomalies. In the brains so far studied the anomalies are predominantly on the left.

6. *Patterns of maturation of the brain.* Studies of patients with early

febrile convulsions and later temporal lobe epilepsy have led to the conclusion that the male brain matures later than the female brain and that the left hemisphere matures later than the right (Taylor 1969). The left planum temporale appears at the 31st week of gestation, whereas the corresponding structure on the right develops 7 to 10 days earlier (Chi, Dooling, and Gilles 1977). In fetal brains gyri and sulci generally develop earlier on the right side (Fontes 1944). Even in infancy dendritic development on the left side in the vicinity of Broca's area lags behind that of its homologue on the right, catching up only later (Scheibel 1984).

7. *Cell death in the developing brain.* In all species studied neurons are formed in excess, and many die when they fail in the competition to form connections (Hamburger and Oppenheim 1982).

8. *Reorganization of the brain after intrauterine lesions.* After surgical ablation of a region of cortex in the fetal monkey, the corresponding cortex of the other side develops a more extensive pattern of bilateral connections than is usually seen (Goldman 1978). Other cortical regions in both the same and the opposite hemisphere increase in size as the result of such lesions (Goldman-Rakic and Rakic 1984).

9. *Hormonal influences on brain structures.* The formation of sexually dimorphic nuclei in the hypothalamus and other structures is dependent on hormonal influences and especially on variations in testosterone level during development (Dörner 1980; Gorski et al. 1980; Pfaff 1966; Raisman and Field 1973; MacLusky and Naftolin 1981; McEwen 1981). Several authors have proposed a relationship between either sex chromosomes or hormones and patterns of cerebral dominance (Netley 1977; Hier and Crowley 1982).

10. *Genetic studies of handedness.* Annett (1978a) has brought evidence that there are individuals in whom cerebral lateralization for speech and handedness is random. Corballis and Morgan (1978) have postulated that asymmetry is an inherent characteristic of the ovum. In twins and their first-degree relatives the rate of lefthandedness is higher than in second-degree relatives (Boklage 1981). This result is consistent with older findings of higher rates of lefthandedness in twins and their singleton relatives than in the general population.

11. *Asymmetries in other species.* Several investigators have demonstrated anatomical and functional asymmetries in other species. (LeMay and Culebras 1972; Nottebohm and Nottebohm 1976; Sherman et al. 1980; Diamond, Dowling, and Johnson 1981).

12. *Chemical asymmetry of the brain.* Serafetinides (1965) found that

hemispheric responses of humans to LSD were asymmetrical. Glick and his coworkers (1979) established the presence of an asymmetry of dopamine content in the rat caudate nucleus, differing in distribution in males and females, and have gone on to establish many other chemical asymmetries.

13. *Evolution of asymmetry.* LeMay and Culebras (1972) have demonstrated asymmetry of the Sylvian fissures in fossil human skulls. Other asymmetries present in modern humans have been found in fossil primate skulls (Holloway and de Lacoste 1982).

14. *Associations of lefthandedness.* We have observed a large group of associations with lefthandedness. Controlled studies have demonstrated a markedly higher frequency of immune disease in strong lefthanders than in strong righthanders (Geschwind and Behan 1982), and this has been confirmed in later studies (Geschwind and Behan 1984; Kolata 1983; M. Kinsbourne and B. Bemporad, personal communication). Elevated rates of lefthandedness have been found in patients with childhood allergies, certain adult immune disorders, and migraine. Older studies documented other associations, such as an elevated rate of lefthandedness among patients with harelip (Tisserand 1944). These observations (as well as others under investigation) have led us to postulate that some of the processes that influence lateralization also affect the development of the immune system and are in turn affected by it, and that processes that disturb cerebral lateralization frequently have widespread effects on other bodily systems.

15. *Relationships of laterality to special talents.* Dyslexics and their families tend to have superior right hemisphere talents (Gordon 1980, 1983). Lefthandedness is much more common in certain groups, for instance, among architects (Peterson and Lansky 1974) and mathematically gifted children (Kolata 1983), who also have a very high rate of allergies.

The lateralization of the nervous system, which has interested clinical neurologists for 120 years, has assumed increasing importance in developmental studies, genetics, linguistics, and psychology. We believe that its significance extends well beyond these disciplines into anthropology, evolution, and comparative zoology, and even into apparently more remote biological fields. As we hope to show, it is relevant to nearly every branch of clinical medicine and to most preclinical disciplines. Lateralization is a central theme in biology and medicine and not simply the esoteric concern of a small number of investigators.

2

Cerebral Dominance: A Brief History of Some Concepts

The concept of lateralization grew out of the discovery in the nineteenth century of cerebral dominance, the superior capacity of each side of the brain to acquire particular skills. The major emphasis over the past 120 years has been on *functional asymmetry*, that is, on the differences in function of the two sides of the brain and of specific regions within them. During that time concepts of cerebral dominance have undergone major changes, and beliefs that were at one time widely accepted have been shown to be incorrect or to require extensive revision.

Broca (1861) was the first to attract widespread attention to cerebral dominance (see figure 2.1). Although predominant use of the right hand had long been recognized, the possibility that manual preference had its origin in the organization of the brain had been considered little or not at all. Broca found that the lesions in his first group of aphasics all lay in delimited regions on the left side. It thus became clear that dominance existed within the human brain; that is, the acquisition of certain abilities appeared to depend on structures located on one side. The special role of the left hemisphere in language seemed to fit in naturally with the preferential use of the right hand by the majority of humans.

The belief that verbal and manual dominance were two aspects of the same function held sway for many years; it was assumed that righthanders had left cerebral dominance for language and that the reverse held for lefthanders. It was soon found, however, that lefthanders sometimes developed aphasia with left hemisphere lesions and that righthanders sometimes became aphasic after right hemisphere lesions. This phenomenon, called *crossed aphasia*, was regarded as a curious exception to the general rule that language and manual dominance shared the same substrate. It was not until after

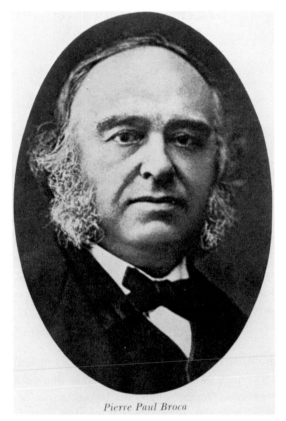

Pierre Paul Broca

Figure 2.1
Pierre Paul Broca, pioneering French physician who brought to the forefront of
nineteenth century neurology the notion that left hemisphere lesions, not right, in-
terfered with normal language function.

World War II that several investigators demonstrated the inaccuracy
of the rule that the same hemisphere was the seat of both language
dominance and hand dominance (Goodglass and Quadfasel 1954;
Zangwill 1960). A new formulation stated that, with rare exceptions,
righthanders had left cerebral dominance for language, whereas 60%
of lefthanders had left dominance and 40% had right dominance. This
formulation, still widely accepted, has also been challenged. It has
been claimed that lefthanders are likely to develop aphasia regardless
of the side of the lesion (Gloning et al. 1969; Satz 1980). This suggests
that strong right cerebral dominance for language either does not
exist or is rare (except after early gross left hemisphere damage) and

that in lefthanders cerebral dominance for language is either left-sided or bilateral. Since even in righthanders extensive left hemisphere damage still leaves some residual language, one might argue that bilateral representation is the rule, ranging, at one extreme, from almost total left dominance, through varying degrees of left superiority, to equal dominance, or, at the other extreme, moderate right-sided dominance (with only rare cases of strong right dominance). Annett (1978b) argues that aphasias with right hemisphere lesions, although still a distinct minority, are far more common than was previously thought. It is clear that any simple assertion of equivalence between dominance for language and dominance for handedness cannot be correct.

Another aspect of the conventional theory, the belief that there was a single dominant hemisphere, grew out of the concept of unitary dominance for language and handedness. The minor (or nondominant) hemisphere was thought to subserve only elementary motor and sensory functions. Those who had dominance divided between the two hemispheres were often regarded as abnormal.

Investigations since World War II have upset the notion of an active, dominant hemisphere and a minor, passive one. Many studies have shown that each hemisphere is usually superior in certain functions (Hécaen 1984; Milner 1973; Benton 1979; Levy 1974). The left hemisphere is usually dominant for language and manual skills; the right hemisphere is more involved in certain spatial and musical abilities, attention, and many aspects of emotion.

The standard theory taught that cerebral dominance was a distinctive feature of humans and of no other species. Only within the past twenty years has this teaching been definitively disproved. Nottebohm and Nottebohm (1976) demonstrated cerebral dominance for song in certain species of birds. Some skeptics believed that avian and human dominance were examples of convergent (that is, independent) evolutionary trends, but the more recent demonstration by Sherman and his coworkers (1980) of right hemisphere dominance for spatial function and emotion in a mammalian species, the rat, has made it likely that functional dominance is widespread in the animal kingdom. Older descriptions of anatomical asymmetries in other species (Larrabee 1906; Kappers, Huber, and Crosby 1936) were generally overlooked but are now joined by more recent discoveries of structural as well as chemical and pharmacological asymmetry in nonhuman animals (LeMay and Geschwind 1975; Kemali, Guiliel-motti, and Gioffre 1980; Diamond 1984; Glick, Jerussi, and Fleisher 1976).

The classical theory also taught that dominance was a property of the cerebral cortex, the latest stage in neurological evolution, which had achieved its greatest complexity in humans. Penfield and Roberts (1959) argued for language dominance in the left thalamus, but this view did not command wide agreement. Milner (1973) demonstrated that left hippocampal removal led to predominantly verbal memory disorders, whereas right-sided ablations led to nonverbal memory difficulties. The participation of subcortical structures in language function has been demonstrated by thalamic stimulation (Ojemann and Ward 1971) and by the finding of aphasias after subcortical lesions (Ciemins 1970; Naeser et al. 1982; Cappa and Vignolo 1979). Asymmetries of function are found even in the brainstem and spinal cord. Several years ago David Cohen pointed out to one of us (NG) that the cardiac autonomic pathways descend predominantly on one side of the brainstem; more recently Faden et al. (1978) found evidence for lateralization of cardiomotor function in the spinal cord.

The classical and contemporary views agree to a great extent on the effects of early and late lesions on dominance. Function often shifts to the opposite hemisphere after unilateral lesions in the first decade of life. Even in adults transfers of this type occur, although much less often. On the average, adult lefthanders and those righthanders with lefthanded first-degree relatives show better recovery from aphasia than unequivocal righthanders (Luria 1970).

One aspect of the older ideas concerning early and late lesions does need to be revised, however. The term "early lesions" is usually applied not only to those occurring in about the first decade of life but also to those occurring prenatally. Yet, as we will discuss later, unilateral lesions and maldevelopments in fetal life, and perhaps even in early postnatal life, will affect lateralization differently from childhood lesions. One must distinguish the effect of disturbances in at least three different stages: fetal (and perhaps early postnatal) life, childhood and adolescence, and adult life.

Despite the vast literature on dominance, few studies have dealt with its neural substrate, its nonbehavioral associations, or its comparative and evolutionary aspects. Older works on the genetics of dominance received some attention, but attempts to account for dominance in terms of anatomical asymmetry aroused little interest.

There were some publications on possible structural associations, for instance, asymmetries of limb length, of fingerprints and other dermatoglyphics, and of other structures, such as hair whorls. Since the existence of dominance in other species was almost universally denied, little consideration was given to the evolution of lateralization. Although developmental disorders such as dyslexia appeared to have a relationship with anomalous dominance, the possible biological mechanisms of these conditions received only occasional comment.

Since the late 1960s there has been a surge of interest in the biology of dominance, reflected in papers on anatomical and chemical asymmetry, structural and functional asymmetries in other species, and biological associations and mechanisms. Many of these studies were reviewed at a meeting in Boston in April, 1983 (Geschwind and Galaburda 1984). Another recent publication deals extensively with studies in nonhuman species (Glick 1985).

It has repeatedly been shown that knowledge of biological mechanism is likely to suggest new approaches for prevention and treatment of disease. The attempt to specify the processes of development opens the way to the use of animal models, although it might on first thought seem impossible to gain useful information about language or developmental dyslexia from experiments in nonhuman species. The brains of all cases of childhood dyslexia so far studied contain cortical regions whose structure is anomalous as a result of disturbances in utero (Galaburda and Kemper 1979; Drake 1968; Galaburda 1984). If dyslexia itself does not occur in the rat or mouse, one can still study neuronal organization and the influences that modify it and thus gain information of potential importance for the prevention and treatment of this disorder. In fact, we have already found two mouse strains that exhibit prenatal unilateral developmental brain lesions comparable to those of the dyslexics. It is also likely, although we will not present the reasons in detail, that the study of brain mechanisms of dominance in other species will lead to a deeper understanding of the underlying principles of language and cognition.

3   A Theory of Lateralization

The simplest theory of lateralization, which is widely accepted, is that patterns of asymmetry are strongly determined genetically. As we will try to demonstrate, this theory has serious shortcomings. Our thesis is that although genes contribute importantly, many influences that lie outside the gene pool of the fetus can alter lateralization patterns. The most powerful factors are variations in the chemical environment in fetal life and, to a lesser extent, in infancy and early childhood. The factors that modify cerebral dominance also influence the development of many other systems, for example, the organs involved in immune response.

It is the intent of this hypothesis to account for the following: (1) Lefthandedness is usually found to be more common in men than women (Oldfield 1971). (2) The developmental disorders of language, speech, cognition, and emotion (such as stuttering, dyslexia, and autism) are strongly male-predominant (Taylor 1974). (3) Females are on the average superior in verbal talents, whereas males tend on the average to be better at spatial functions (Maccoby and Jacklin 1974; Wittig and Petersen 1979). (4) Lefthanders of both sexes and those with learning disabilities often exhibit superior right hemisphere functions (Gordon 1980, 1983; Peterson and Lansky 1974). (5) Lefthandedness and ambidexterity are more frequent in the developmental disorders of childhood (Hécaen 1984; Diehl 1958; Porac and Coren 1981). (6) Certain diseases, such as immune disorders, are more common in nonrighthanders (Geschwind and Behan 1982, 1984).

The human brain is asymmetrical even in fetal life, with a pattern resembling that seen in adult life, for example, a right Sylvian fissure angled up more at its posterior end than the left (LeMay and Culebras 1972) and a larger left planum temporale (Wada, Clarke, and Hamm

1975; Witelson and Pallie 1973; Chi, Dooling, and Gilles 1977; Teszner et al. 1972). In fetal brains the gyral and sulcal patterns develop earlier on the right side (Fontes 1944). These findings are compatible with the concept that the fundamental pattern of the brain usually includes strong asymmetries favoring the structures around the left Sylvian fissure. There is probably some influence that slows the growth of parts of the left hemisphere so that, for reasons to be given, the corresponding regions on the right develop relatively more rapidly. On the basis of the higher frequency of lefthandedness and of learning disorders in males, it has been postulated that this influence is related to male sex, for instance, to testosterone or some factor related to it. H-Y antigen, to be discussed later, is normally present only in male fetuses, but this cannot be the exclusive male-related factor, since, if it were, the similar (although less marked) effects in females could not be accounted for. Both male and female fetuses are exposed to maternal and placental hormones. Once the male testes develop, the titer of testosterone rises to high levels. The formation of the testes and the secretion of testosterone are essential to the development of most of the features that differentiate males from females in most species. The female fetus is also exposed to testosterone, although in lower quantities. Factors that determine sensitivity to testosterone, or other male-related influences, will be important in both sexes. Both sexes are exposed to high levels of progesterone, which may have masculinizing effects on female fetuses at certain stages of development (Meyer-Bahlburg and Ehrhardt 1980).

The male-related influence thus acts to alter the expression of certain genes that play an important role in neural development. Many other influences could act on these genes, of course, but some male-related factor must be of special importance.

Major effects of testosterone on neural development have been demonstrated in many studies, mostly in the rat, on the factors determining gender-specific sexual characteristics (such as the cyclic release of gonadotropins in the female) and behavior. Testosterone induces a change in the structure of specific nuclei in the hypothalamus and limbic system. Sex hormone receptors are widely distributed in many neural and nonneural tissues (Stumpf et al. 1976) and are found in the cortex of the newborn rat (gestationally equivalent to the human fetus in late pregnancy). Recently they have been found in the cortex of the infant monkey as well, especially in association areas (P.S. Goldman-Rakic, personal communication).

If some factor delays the growth of portions of the left hemisphere, changes must take place in other regions (particularly the homologous regions in the opposite hemisphere and unaffected ones in the same hemisphere) as a result of mechanisms that have been studied in recent years. Many neurons in the fetal nervous system die in utero and, in the rat, in the early postnatal period as well. Recent data suggest that postnatal cell death also occurs in humans (Huttenlocher 1979). Although all the factors involved in cell death have not been specified, it is known that a neuron is more likely to die if it fails to establish connections. Goldman (1978) has studied the changes in the pattern of connections that follow intrauterine lesions of one frontal cortex in the monkey. Normally each frontal cortex projects primarily to the ipsilateral thalamus and caudate nucleus. After an intrauterine lesion of one frontal cortex the intact homologous cortex on the opposite side not only forms the usual ipsilateral connections but also develops a large number of connections with the caudate nucleus and thalamus on the side of the lesioned cortex. It has also been shown that after ablation of a cortical area in intrauterine life other cortical regions are found in later life to be larger than normal (Goldman-Rakic and Rakic 1984). The homologous area on the side opposite the lesion and areas adjacent to the one lesioned are likely to show such an increase in size. This enlargement is presumably the result of death of fewer neurons and possibly of greater size of neurons in the intact regions of cortex because neurons in the lesioned area have been taken out of the competition for targets. A delay in development of some cortical regions on the left side should lead to the same effects; that is, it should favor growth of cortical regions on the opposite side and of unaffected regions on the same side. The larger of two areas will probably have not only more surviving cells but also more extensive bilateral connections, a feature that may well be characteristic of dominant regions.

The hypothesis suggests that growth retardation will generally be more marked in certain left hemisphere regions in men, who will therefore show on the average a greater degree of shift to right-hemisphere participation in handedness and language and will therefore more likely have augmented right hemisphere skills. In addition, they may have elevated skills related to unaffected regions on the left. Excessive delays caused by male-related factors will be more common in men. In some cases there will be markedly delayed neuronal migration and/or abnormal neuronal assembly, especially in left hemisphere language regions; for example, there will be disrupted cortical architecture and neurons in abnormal locations. Regions of disordered cytoarchitecture or disturbed neuronal migration confined to the left hemisphere have been found in the brains of several childhood dyslexics. The higher rate of such disruptions of cortical architecture in the left speech regions in men accounts for the greater rate of developmental learning disorders in boys.

The effect of testosterone may depend either on the level of the free hormone (that is, not bound to sex-hormone-binding globulin) or on tissue sensitivity. Thus, some female fetuses in whom sensitivity is high will also manifest excessive testosterone effects. Progesterone effects that are not the result of exogenously administered hormone may also reflect individual differences in sensitivity.

Testosterone also affects the growth of many other tissues. In particular, it retards the growth of structures involved in immunity, such as the bursa of Fabricius in the chick embryo (Warner, Szenberg, and Burnet 1962) and the thymus gland in the rat postnatally (Frey-Wettstein and Craddock 1970). Recent experiments in the rabbit by Behan (P. Behan, personal communication) are consistent with similar retarding effects on the fetal thymus. Thus, when testosterone effects on the brain are most marked, development of the immune system may be altered, heightening susceptibility to later immune disorders. It might be argued that this mechanism would lead to a higher rate of immune disorders in males. There is, however, another effect that protects males, especially in the postpubertal period. Testosterone suppresses the thymus even in adult life (Frey-Wettstein and Craddock 1970; Wasi and Block 1961), so that thymic involution after puberty is more pronounced in males. In the New Zealand Black-White, F1 hybrid mouse (NZB/W) model the milder course of disease in the male depends on the presence of testosterone (Talal 1977a). This hypothesis is compatible with the fact that certain autoimmune disorders such as lupus erythematosus and myasthenia are most frequent in young females (that is, when testosterone effects are at a minimum) and that the proportion of male cases rises with age, as testosterone effects decline. We have also found that atopic disorders (for example, asthma, eczema, and hay fever) are more frequent in lefthanders. The fact that atopic disorders are more common in males in childhood (before the pubertal rise in testosterone) but more common in females after puberty (Crawford and Beldham 1976) is also compatible with this hypothesis.

The relationship between testosterone and immunity is probably a very close one. Ivanyi (1978) has shown that several loci in the major histocompatibility complex of the mouse, whose importance in immune mechanisms is established, also code for various aspects of the production and metabolism of testosterone and for expression of the H-Y antigen on the thymus. These and other relationships between sex hormones and immunity will be detailed later. Whether or not the specific hypothesis proposed here is the correct one (and, even if basically correct, it will certainly undergo major modification), it seems clear that there is an intimate relationship among sex hormones, immunity, and laterality.

Asymmetrical development is a property not only of the cortex but also of many other parts of the nervous system and of other organs. The factors that influence cortical asymmetry and the structures of the immune system will also modify development—and, in particular, asymmetrical development—in other systems. We will discuss in particular the evidence for asymmetry in neural crest migrations and will raise the possibility that some changes in neural structures are secondary to effects on the neural crest. It has been shown that influences acting in utero or in very early postnatal life may permanently alter certain metabolic systems; we will raise the possibility that such alterations may accompany shifts in dominance. We will also suggest that such intrauterine influences may modify susceptibility to certain diseases in later life, even in old age. In particular, regions whose development is disturbed in fetal life may be especially susceptible to later immune or infectious attack.

It should be stressed that frank lefthanders constitute only one easily identifiable group with an anomalous (nonstandard) pattern of dominance. We postulate that the basic pattern of the brain is one with strong left hemisphere asymmetry for the substrates of language and handedness. Influences that delay left hemisphere growth thus tend to create brains in which the normal asymmetry of these regions is diminished, so that the corresponding areas on the two sides are more symmetrical. The group with symmetrical brains should manifest a phenomenon postulated by Annett (1978a), namely, random dominance. Many individuals subjected to left hemisphere delays will have random handedness, and thus roughly as many will be righthanded as lefthanded. Lefthanders will therefore constitute only a fraction of the anomalous dominance group (our guess is about one-third), which includes perhaps 30% of the population.

There is another reason why lefthandedness will not be present in many individuals in whom growth of the cortex has been delayed. There is no reason to assume that the delaying effect will be present all through gestation. It is likely that the observed dominance patterns of cortical regions will differ depending on the exact period, or periods, in pregnancy in which the effects of testosterone or related factors are elevated. In some cases the as yet unknown substrate of handedness may have developed during a period in which there is no significant retarding effect. A delaying influence appearing later (for instance, a subsequent rise in testosterone levels or sensitivity) may slow the formation of later-developing regions (for instance, the temporal speech area). If this type of pattern occurred frequently, one might find anomalous dominance for language more often than for handedness.

The earlier development of the right hemisphere implies that it will be less subject to disrupting influences. As a result, we expect that disturbances in cytoarchitectonic structure will be less frequent on the right than on the left. In addition, early influences that disturb the development of the right hemisphere will often persist through later periods and thus have more widespread effects. Right hemisphere retardation may therefore often be accompanied by left hemisphere delay, but in many cases retardation of left-sided development will follow normal development of the right side. In the latter case the right-sided areas may, after the period of cell death, be larger than normal.

In the chapters to follow we will present these findings in more detail and will discuss their implications, namely, that although genetic factors must play a large role, nongenetic factors will greatly influence the development of dominance. We will also consider implications for giftedness. Since the influences that produce delays in the left hemisphere will lead to final greater extent of other cortical regions, this process may be a mechanism of giftedness. This accounts for the elevated level of nonrighthanders in architecture and certain other occupations. Frank neuronal migration disorders may thus be not only a pathology of defect but also a "pathology of superiority" that explains the presence of very high talents in many cases of autism, dyslexia, and stuttering and the common occurrence of superior right hemisphere functions in dyslexics and their families. Finally we will address the question of the fundamental mechanisms by which asymmetrical structures are formed and will consider the possibility that certain common mechanisms may be at play in both the plant and the animal kingdoms.

4   Normal Development of the Brain

Cerebral asymmetry is found even during early fetal life. Before we consider the processes that lead to lateralization, it will be helpful to review the stages of normal cortical development.

Although many earlier descriptions of brain development were derived from observations on the human fetus, recent research has been carried out primarily on experimental animals. Thus, although the general outlines of the schedules and patterns of human cerebral development are known, certain details can be drawn only by inference from studies in other species.

No neuron is formed in the cortex itself. All cortical neurons are generated in the neural tube, from which they migrate to their future locations. The development of neural structures proceeds in an orderly sequence: (1) *neural induction* (Saxen and Toivonen 1962), that is, formation of the primitive neural elements; (2) *differentiation of the neural plate* (Jacobson 1959); (3) *formation of the neural tube* (Karfunkel 1974), which will give rise to the central nervous system; (4) *formation of the neural crest* (Weston 1970; LeDouarin 1982), dorsal to the neural tube, from which cells will migrate to form peripheral sensory and autonomic ganglia and other derivatives (for instance, certain endocrine glands, some components of the thymus, thyroid, and parathyroid glands, some elements of the musculoskeletal system, nearly all pigmented cells of the skin and other structures, and the skin and bones of the face); (5) *formation of germinal zones* (Jacobson 1978), which generate neuronal and glial precursors; (6) *cell migration* (Marin-Padilla 1970), during which neuronal and glial elements will travel to their permanent locations; (7) *cellular differentiation and maturation* (Jacobson 1978), during which neurons in their final locations grow and establish connections; (8) *massive neuronal death and axonal attrition* (Cowan 1973) (although cell death probably occurs to some extent during each stage and continues even into the postnatal period).

In the first weeks of fetal development there is rapid replication of DNA. After the later phase of DNA replication cells move toward the lumen of the neural tube to form the *ventricular germinal zone* (also known as the *subependymal zone, subependymal cell plate,* or *ependymal cell layer),* in which cells proliferate. The neural tube is thus differentiated into a *germinal zone* and a cell-free *marginal zone.* It is possible later to distinguish an *intermediate zone,* lying between the ventricular and marginal zones, which contains postmitotic cells moving toward the pial surface. The *subventricular zone,* which contains proliferating glia and some special classes of neurons, appears as an additional germinal zone between the ventricular and intermediate zones. Mitosis takes place only in the germinal zones, and cells migrate only after the completion of mitosis. Every neuron found in the cortex of a mature animal migrated in fetal life from the neural tube to its final location.

During the period of proliferation the generation of cells obeys the following rules: (1) there are spatial and temporal gradients; (2) cells destined to populate separate architectonic zones have separate origins; (3) cells are produced in a specific sequence of sizes—first large neurons, then intermediate-sized neurons, and finally small neurons; (4) glia destined for a given region of the brain tend to originate after neurons; and (5) phylogenetically older parts of the brain tend to arise earlier in ontogeny.

The cellular migration that follows proliferation occurs in waves. During this stage the cortical mantle begins to form at the junction of the intermediate and marginal zones, and it increases in thickness with each successive wave of arriving neurons and glia. The cortical plate is soon differentiated into a deeper layer containing more mature cells that have arrived at an earlier period and a more superficial layer containing later-arriving, more immature neurons. Those cells that arrive later must thus move through the layers already formed in order to reach the outer surface. The process is even more complex; nerve cells seem to be in constant movement, so that they may pass through their eventual permanent sites and then return to them. The ventricular zone becomes thinner as it continues to lose cells during the course of migration, and the two-layer cortical plate thickens.

The production of neurons and the consolidation of the ventricular zone begin at around the 6th week of gestation. The first wave of migration to the cortical plate and its first differentiation take place between the 6th and 8th weeks. The subventricular zone is formed between the 8th and 10th weeks. From the 11th to the 13th weeks the cortical plate differentiates into two layers, the thickening of which continues through the end of the 15th week. Cellular migration to the cortex is completed between the 6th and 8th fetal months.

The stage of cell differentiation, especially in the deeper layers, begins roughly during the 16th week, before cell migration to the superficial layers is completed, and continues well into the postnatal period. During this stage neurons grow, develop their dendrites and axons, and establish synaptic contacts. Cortical maturation also involves *myelogenesis,* which takes place in an orderly, regionalized fashion; it begins in the cortex before birth and continues well into adult life, the myelination of the tangential intracortical layers taking place very late. The great postnatal increase in brain weight is largely the result of accumulation of myelin. Myelination, like cellular proliferation and migration, generally occurs earlier in phylogenetically older regions; large neurons with long axons (present mostly in the deeper layers) myelinate before small neurons with short axons.

As will be discussed in greater detail later, the neuronal migration and assembly may be modified by circulating sex hormones. Estrogens enhance cortical maturation and myelogenesis in the rat (Heim and Timiras 1963; Curry and Heim 1966), whereas androgens interfere with this estrogen effect (Toran-Allerand 1978) in vitro and in vivo. Sexual dimorphism in neural organization can result from the differential effects of gonadal hormones during the stage of cell maturation (Toran-Allerand 1978), but sex hormones may also affect the proliferation and migration of neurons. At the time in the early postnatal period in which the maximum number of estradiol receptors and peak estradiol levels are found in the rodent brain, there is also intense sprouting of neurites and myelination of axons. It is important to stress that these hormonal effects are limited to brain areas having the appropriate hormone receptors and enzymes and to critical periods during which the receptors are sensitive to the effects of the particular hormone.

A crucial factor in cortical development, which helps to match the number of presynaptic neurons with available synaptic sites, is the process of cell death, which reduces the great excess of neurons produced in fetal life. Cell death can be enhanced experimentally; for example, a focal lesion placed at a critical time decreases the number of postsynaptic sites and thus leads to increased death of neurons projecting to that structure. The process is graded; reduction of the number of appropriate synaptic sites results in an increased rate of cell death, whereas the experimental addition of postsynaptic sites can diminish it. The absolute number of available postsynaptic sites only partly determines which cells will die; there appear to be specific recognition properties that place some cells at an advantage in establishing connections. It is likely, however, that of two presynaptic axons having equal affinity for the postsynaptic site, the one arriving first has a greater chance of surviving. Thus, a neuronal system that develops quickly, or whose axons grow more rapidly, comes to predominate over slower competing systems. When differences in developmental rate are affected by the numbers of receptors for hormones or other substances, the relative extent of cell death in competing presynaptic systems may come under hormonal regulation during critical periods.

The lack of a given postsynaptic site need not lead to the loss of the presynaptic cell if that cell can establish connections elsewhere (Goldman and Galkin 1978; Innocenti 1981). The reshaping of neuronal circuits, because of availability of alternative postsynaptic sites, has been shown by the placement of lesions during development. These experiments reveal the patterns of cell death resulting from the removal of postsynaptic sites, the rerouting of presynaptic axons to other available postsynaptic sites, and the invasion of other axons of postsynaptic sites left vacant by the loss of neurons destroyed by the lesion. When a cortical visual area in the cat that normally receives transcallosal axons is lesioned in early life, there is a marked loss of neurons in the appropriate contralateral cortex (Innocenti 1981); some of the contralateral neurons do survive, however, because their axons change their trajectories and establish ipsilateral connections. Reorganization of connections may occur across the midline. Thus, unilateral collicular lesions in hamsters increase projections to the contralateral colliculus (Schneider 1981), and contralateral projections from frontal cortex to thalamus are enhanced when the ipsilateral frontal cortex is lesioned (Goldman 1979). It is likely that the striking findings in these experiments reflect mechanisms of adaptation to normal variations in the environment of the growing brain, which can alter the availability and location of postsynaptic sites in the developing nervous system.

5   Asymmetry of the Human Brain

In this chapter we will discuss the advantages of an asymmetrical nervous system, summarize some of the known anatomical asymmetries found in the human at a gross and cytoarchitectonic level, and present the available data on their development. We will cite studies in nonhuman species when relevant, but we reserve a fuller discussion of animal asymmetries for chapter 6.

5.1 The Advantages of a Lateralized Brain

The common belief that most animals are symmetrical is far from true. An axis of external symmetry is usually present, but internal asymmetry is probably the rule. It was long believed that the brain was symmetrical in both humans and other species. It is likely, however, that every vertebrate species will be shown to have an asymmetrical nervous system, and, as will be pointed out later, the same is probably true for invertebrates. Surprisingly, even single-celled organisms are commonly asymmetrical. It is possible, however, that the most complex nervous systems show the most elaborate patterns of asymmetrical function. Humans are not unique in the possession of lateralized functions, but they may well be endowed with the most extensively asymmetrical brains.

The ability to learn and to adapt to changing environments has played a major role in the survival of higher animals. The human race, which survives in almost any ecological niche, owes its biological success primarily to its brain, and cerebral dominance must have contributed heavily to human adaptive capacities.

It may appear strange that dominance has increasingly won out over duplication, but the advantages of redundancy are not as great as they might at first appear to be. The cat's superior recovery from hemiplegia is of little advantage in the wild, since a few days or even a few hours of disability mean almost certain death. By contrast, lateral specialization makes possible a larger complement of talents that may be useful in survival. Furthermore, the more functions represented in the brain the greater the diversity of endowment within the species, so that some members will survive almost any new threat. The modification of dominance by intrauterine environmental changes increases diversity to a far greater extent than a rigid genetic mechanism would allow.

It might be argued that dominance could be present even in the absence of structural asymmetry. An example may be the HVc nucleus of the songbird (Nottebohm and Arnold 1976), which does not differ in size on the two sides despite unilateral dominance for song. Even in the songbird there is a small but significant difference in the size of the twelfth-nerve nucleus (which is about 15% larger on the left dominant side in the chaffinch). However, we suspect that, at least in mammals, anatomical asymmetry will be the rule. At the very least, one would expect an asymmetrical pattern of connections so that each side could control different functions. A pattern that may well be common will be that of a unilaterally larger area with more extensive bilateral outputs and inputs than the opposite region.

In chapter 19 we will discuss some of the known causes of anatomical asymmetry and present hypotheses regarding other possible mechanisms. Several different types of process may contribute to the neural asymmetries of higher animals.

5.2 Gross Anatomical Asymmetries

Ever since Broca discovered the functional lateralization of the human brain, structural asymmetries have been sought to explain left hemisphere specialization for language. Some early articles described asymmetries of hemispheric length, weight, or total surface area, but these were often very small or inconsistent (Rey 1885). Later authors did find reproducible asymmetries (Pfeifer 1936; Economo and Horn 1930; Fukui 1934; Kakeshita 1925), but their publications were generally neglected. In 1962 von Bonin dismissed the earlier work as uncontrolled or lacking in adequate statistical support and concluded that minor anatomical asymmetries were present in the brain that could not account for the dramatic functional asymmetries. Geschwind and Levitsky (1968) reinvestigated this question and found a

Table 5.1
Anatomical asymmetries in the human brain

Structure	Righthanders (RH)				Lefthanders (LH)				Comments
	N	L>	L=R	R>	N	L>	L=R	R>	
Frontal lobe (Gundara and Zivanovic 1968)	297	28	23	49	...	...	...	...	Petalia in East African skulls; no handedness; percentages
Frontal lobe (Lemay 1976)	174	9	21	70	49	21	40	39	Width by CT scan; adults and children; percentages
Frontal lobe (Lemay 1976)	206	7	63	30	58	21	60	19	Petalia by CT scan; adults and children; percentages
Frontal lobe (LeMay 1977)	...	...	...	...	39	18	29	53	CT width in nonfamilial lefthanders; percentages
Frontal lobe	...	...	...	...	39	28	21	51	CT petalia in nonfamilial lefthanders; percentages
Frontal lobe	...	...	...	...	41	41	25	34	CT petalia in familial lefthanders; percentages
Frontal lobe (Chui and Damasio 1980)	50	8	56	36	25	16	56	28	CT petalia; percentages; LH includes ambidextrous
Frontal lobe (Holloway 1980)	5	1	0	4	...	...	...	...	Petalia in endocasts of Solo Man: no handedness
Frontal lobe (Weinberger et al. 1982)	40	...	...	80	...	...	...	...	Volume of frontal lobe from Yakovlev Collection; adults, children, and infants; no handedness; percentages

					Description
Inferior frontal gyrus (Wada, Clarke, and Hamm 1975)	100	21.5	⋮	...	⋮	26.7	Mean convexity area in cm² of opercular portion; adults; no handedness
	85	21.7	...	25.8	Mean convexity area in cm² of opercular portion; infants and fetuses; no handedness
Inferior frontal gyrus (Galaburda 1980)	102	26	61	13	Brains with extra sulcus in pars opercularis; adults and children; no handedness; percentages
Inferior frontal gyrus (Nikkuni et al. 1981)	54	44	39	17	Convexity area in cm² of pars opercularis and pars triangularis; no handedness; adults
	10	66	17	17	Children
	4	0	100	0	Infants
Inferior frontal gyrus (Falzi, Perrone, and Vignolo 1982)	12	8	1	3	Total area of frontal operculum
Inferior frontal gyrus (Galaburda 1980)	10	6	3	1	Total volume of opercular architectonic area 44; adults and children; no handedness
Temporal lobe (Fukui 1934)	75	75	12	13	Area of PT; no handedness; percentages
Temporal lobe (Geschwind and Levitsky 1968)	100	65	24	11	Length of lateral edge of PT; adults; no handedness; percentages
Temporal lobe (Teszner et al. 1972)	100	75	12.5	12.5	Area of PT; adults; no handedness; percentages

Table 5.1
(continued)

Structure	N	Righthanders (RH)			Lefthanders (LH)				Comments
		L>	L=R	R>	N	L>	L=R	R>	
Temporal lobe (Witelson Pallie 1973)	16	81	...	...	...	...	...	...	Length of PT; no handedness; percentages; adults
	14	66	...	...	...	...	...	...	Infants
	16	69	0	31	...	...	...	...	Area of PT; no handedness; percentages; adults
	14	79	...	...	...	...	...	...	Infants
Temporal lobe (Wada, Clarke, and Hamm 1975)	100	82	8	10	...	...	...	...	Area of PT; no handedness; percentages; adults
	100	56	32	12	...	...	...	...	Infants
Temporal lobe (Rubens, Mahowald, and Hutton 1976)	21	67	...	...	...	...	...	...	Length of PT; adults; no handedness; percentages
Temporal lobe (Campain and Minckler 1976)	30	3	47	50	...	...	...	...	Percentages with more than one gyrus of Heschl; adults and children; no handedness
Temporal lobe (Kopp et al. 1977)	103	77	1	22	...	...	...	...	Area of PT; no handedness; percentages
Temporal lobe (Nikkuni et al. 1981)	54	83	9	7	...	...	...	...	Area of PT; no handedness; percentages; adults
	10	70	20	10	...	...	...	...	Children
	4	50	50	0	...	...	...	...	Infants

									Area of PT
Temporal lobe (Falzi, Perrone, and Vignolo 1982)	12	10	...	2	...	...	...	...	Area of PT
Temporal lobe (Galaburda, Sanides, and Geschwind 1978)	4	3	1	...	...	...	...	...	Volume of architectonic area Tpt; adults and children; no handedness
Occipital lobe (Gundara and Zivanovic 1968)	297	52	24	24	...	...	...	...	Petalia in East African skulls; no handedness; percentages
Occipital lobe (LeMay 1976)	150	64	20	16	50	22	32	16	Width by CT scan; adults and children; percentages
	269	69	22	9	62	56	24	20	Petalia by CT scan; adults and children; percentages
	...	...	...	...	40	37	39	24	Width by CT scan; adults and children; percentages; familial lefthandedness
	...	...	...	...	37	59	22	19	No familial lefthandedness
	...	...	...	...	41	29	32	39	Petalia by CT scan; adults and children; percentages; familial lefthandedness
	...	...	...	...	39	59	15	26	No familial lefthandedness
Occipital lobe (Chui and Damasio 1980)	50	60	20	20	25	44	36	20	CT petalia; percentages; LH includes ambidextrous
Occipital lobe (Holloway 1980)	5	4	1	0	...	...	...	...	Petalia in endocasts of Solo Man; no handedness

Table 5.1
(continued)

Structure	N	Righthanders (RH)				Lefthanders (LH)			Comments
		L>	L=R	R>	N	L>	L=R	R>	
Occipital lobe (Weinberger 1982)	40	...	...	80	...	...	...	...	Volume of occipital lobe from Yakovlev Collection; adults, children, infants; no handedness; percentages
Occipital horn (McRae, Branch, and Milner 1968)	87	60	30	10	13	38	31	31	Length by PEG; percentages
Occipital horn	75	39	44	17	...	...	...	...	Length by PEG; children, some with neurological abnormalities; no handedness; percentages
Parietal lobe (Eidelberg and Galaburda 1984)	8	5	1	2	...	...	...	...	Volume of architectonic area PG; direct correlation with asymmetry in PT; adults and children; no handedness
Sylvian fissure (LeMay and Culebras 1972)	44	5	9	86	18	11	72	17	Height of posterior and of Sylvian fissure on carotid A-grams; adults and children; percentages
Sylvian fissure (Hochberg and LeMay 1975)	100	7	26	67	28	7	71	22	Height of posterior and Sylvian fissure on carotid A-grams; adults and children; percentages
Sylvian fissure (Rubens, Mahowald, and Hutton 1976)	36	75	...	...	...	...	...	...	Length of Sylvian fissure; adults; no handedness; percentages

Sylvian fissure (Yeni-Komshian and Benson 1976)	25	84	0	16	...	...	...	...	Length of Sylvian fissure; no handedness; percentages
Sylvian fissure (Ratcliff et al. 1980)	38	21	21	58	20	15	35	50	Height of posterior and of Sylvian fissure on carotid A-grams; percentages
Thalamus (Eidelberg and Galaburda 1982)	9	8	0	1	...	...	...	...	Volume of nucleus lateralis posterior; adults and children; no handedness
Bulbar pyramids (Kertesz and Geschwind 1971)	123	73	10	17	7	88	0	14	Side from which decussation is higher in the brain stem; adults and children; percentages

Abbreviations: *CT*, computer-assisted tomography; *PT*, planum temporale; *PEG*, pneumoencephalogram; *A-gram*, arteriogram

striking asymmetry of the portion of the upper surface of the temporal lobe lying behind the gyrus of Heschl. Their findings have been
confirmed repeatedly, and other human brain asymmetries have
been described. A summary of these lateral differences is presented in
table 5.1.

The first consistently found asymmetry in the human brain was
described almost simultaneously by Cunningham (1892) in Ireland
and by Eberstaller (1884) in Germany. They found the Sylvian fissures
to be asymmetrical at the posterior end (the Sylvian point at which
the middle cerebral artery exits from the Sylvian fossa). The right
fissure curls upward posteriorly and thus ends in a higher position
than the left, an asymmetry that can be seen in cerebral arteriograms
and in postmortem specimens (LeMay and Culebras 1972) (see
figures 5.1, 5.2, 5.3). The pattern of this asymmetry varies with hand-

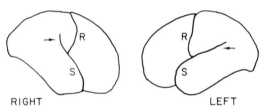

RIGHT   LEFT

Figure 5.1
Standard asymmetry of the Sylvian fissures (arrows). The shorter, upwardly curved
right fissure points to a smaller development of the temporal and parietal opercula
on that side.

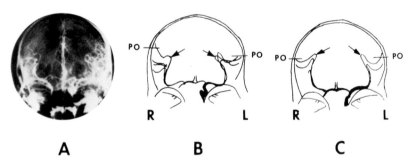

A   B   C

Figure 5.2
Standard asymmetry of the Sylvian fissues (A and B) and symmetrical case (C) as
seen on cerebral arteriography (LeMay and Culebras 1972). The more acute angle of
the left middle cerebral artery branches (B, right arrow) accommodates the lower-
lying left parietal operculum (PO). Also note that the symmetrical case illustrates
bilaterally the standard left-sided pattern. Reprinted by permission of the *New
England Journal of Medicine* 287:168–170, 1972.

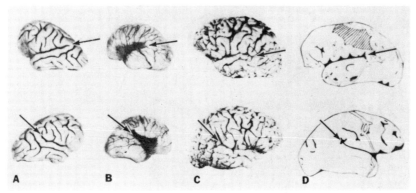

A   B   C   D

Figure 5.3
Asymmetry of the Sylvian fissures exhibited in the orangutan (*A*), the human fetus
(*B*), the human adult (*C*), and a Neanderthal endocast (*D*) (LeMay 1984). Irrespective
of the detailed functional phenotypes accompanying these homologous structural
asymmetries, the observation supports the notion of a long biologically based phy-
logenetic history for cerebral lateralization. Reprinted by permission of the author
and Harvard University Press.

edness (Hochberg and LeMay 1975). As can be seen in table 5.1, a bias
toward a higher right sylvian fissure is much stronger among self-
described righthanders than among lefthanders.

It was also demonstrated quite early that the left Sylvian fissure
is usually longer than the right, suggesting that the temporal and
parietal opercula, which make up the floor and the roof of the Sylvian
fossa, are larger on the left than on the right. The fact that the posterior temporal operculum is larger on the left side was originally
shown by Pfeifer (1936), who pointed out that the planum temporale
was larger on the left side (see figures 5.4, 5.5). Subsequently, Geschwind and Levitsky (1968) showed in 100 adult human brains that
the left planum was usually larger, a result since confirmed by several
other investigators (Wada, Clarke, and Hamm 1975; Witelson and
Pallie 1973; Teszner et al. 1972; Kopp et al. 1977). Meyer (1950)
showed that the planum temporale is involved in language functions;
it is, in fact, the extension on the upper surface of the temporal lobe of
the speech area of Wernicke.

Two features of these data are potentially important. First, asymmetry is the rule in the planum, being evident in at least three-
quarters of the brains studied in all series. Second, the magnitude of
the asymmetry is often dramatic, so that the left planum is sometimes
ten times larger than the right. Although asymmetries of this mag-

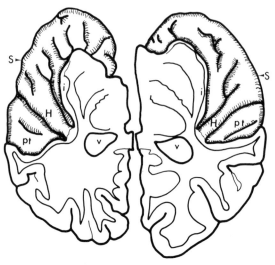

Figure 5.4
Standard asymmetry of the planum temporale (*pt*), the roughly triangular region lying posterior (inferior in the diagram) to the transverse auditory gyrus of Heschl (*H*) and bound laterally by the Sylvian fissure (*S*). This pattern of asymmetry is seen in approximately two-thirds of normal human brains. Other abbreviations: *i*, insula; *v*, lateral ventricle.

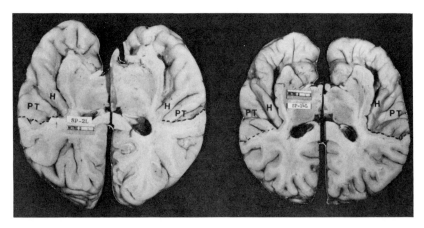

Figure 5.5
Symmetry and asymmetry in the human planum temporale (*PT*). Two observations characterize these cases: (1) when the brain is symmetrical in this region, both plana tend to be relatively large (that is, the standard left planum pattern is preserved bilaterally); (2) the splenium of the corpus callosum (cut in the midline of the photographs) appears to be thicker in the symmetrical cases.

nitude may be seen in subcortical structures of other species, as in the habenular nucleus of the lamprey (Kappers, Huber, and Crosby 1936), no nonhuman species yet studied has shown such a degree of lateral disparity in the cortex.

Pfeifer also pointed out that a second transverse gyrus was more likely to be found on the right than on the left, a result confirmed by later authors (Beck 1955; Campain and Minckler 1976). Even in fetal life the right planum, which develops earlier than the left, is more likely to have two transverse gyri (Chi, Dooling, and Gilles 1977).

Broca (1863) was the first to give a detailed description of the anterior horizontal and ascending limbs of the Sylvian fissure, located in the opercular portion of the frontal lobe. The horizontal limb makes up the rostral boundary of the pars triangularis, and the ascending limb makes up the caudal boundary. Eberstaller (1884) noted that the ascending Sylvian limb was more often branched on the left than on the right. This suggested that the left frontal opercular region, which makes up part of Broca's speech area, was more infolded and thus contained more cortex than the corresponding region on the right. In a study of brains of righthanders Falzi, Perrone, and Vignolo (1982) have found an average of 22% more infolded cortex in the left than in the right frontal operculum.

McRae, Branch, and Milner (1968) showed that in pneumoencephalograms of righthanders the occipital horn of the left lateral ventricle is usually longer than that of the right one, whereas in lefthanders the occipital horn asymmetry is nearly equally distributed between the right and left sides. Similar asymmetries in the occipital horns have been demonstrated by the use of computerized tomography (CT).

The petalias are another group of anatomical asymmetries that can be seen in modern and fossil skulls and in CT scans. A petalia is a more marked indentation in the inner table of the skull on one side that results from the greater protrusion of the adjacent cerebral lobe on that side than on the other (figure 5.6; see also figure 6.1). LeMay (1977) has shown in righthanded individuals a predominance of left occipital petalia: a wider and/or longer occipital lobe is found nearly four times more often on the left than on the right, and a wider and/or longer frontal lobe is found almost nine times more frequently on the right than on the left. In lefthanded subjects the distribution is much more symmetrical. All investigators agree that the left occipital lobe is usually wider or longer, but there is disagreement regarding the exact

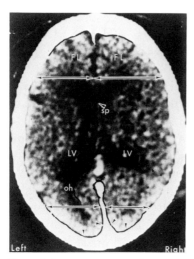

Figure 5.6
Standard asymmetry of the human cerebral hemispheres as seen by computer-assisted tomography (Galaburda et al. 1978). This pattern consists of a broader right frontal lobe (*FL*, upper arrows) and a broader and longer (lower arrows and arrowheads, respectively) left occipital lobe. Other abbreviations: *sp*, septum pellucidum; *LV*, lateral ventricle; *oh*, occipital horn of LV. Copyright 1978 by the AAAS.

statistics and whether the distribution varies with handedness. There is also some disagreement on whether the right frontal lobe is usually the larger one. Thus, the one lobar asymmetry whose existence is generally agreed to is that of the left occipital region. The reasons for the disagreements are still unclear. They may reflect differences in radiological technique or methods of measurement, in selection of subjects (one study used children with epilepsy as normal controls, which is probably not justified), or in criteria for handedness.

Another question is how many independent petalias exist. In a study of East African skulls Gundara and Zivanovic (1968) found not only a predominance of right frontal and left occipital petalias but also a predominance of left parietal petalia that appears to be independent of the occipital petalia. We will not pursue these issues further here; we believe that they will be resolved only by further studies and by further anatomical investigations of brains obtained at postmortem.

These studies nevertheless raise an issue of theoretical importance: Are certain asymmetries linked, or are they independent? Assume, for example, that one particular asymmetry in favor of the left side occurs in 80% of brains, whereas another asymmetry in favor of the right side is also found in 80%. If the two asymmetries were linked, as many as 80% of brains might be expected to show both. If they are independent, both should occur together in 64%. If they are negatively related, they would still cooccur in not less than 60% of cases. Very large samples would be needed to distinguish the three cases. In the study by Gundara and Zivanovic the frequencies of the eight possible combinations of occipital, frontal, and parietal petalias are consistent with independent occurrence of the various asymmetries.

The larger the number of independent asymmetries the greater the possible diversity of the population. In any case the data should be ascertained, since they will place important constraints on any theory.

There is a spectrum of degrees of human cerebral asymmetry. Although the left planum may be many times larger than the right, equally dramatic examples of right-sided planum superiority are uncommon; moreover, in about 25% of cases there is little difference between the sides. The distribution observed for the planum—about 65% favoring the left and about 35% roughly equal or favoring the right—reappears in relation to other asymmetries. It is conceivable that the figure of 35% may represent the proportion of the population with anomalous dominance for language, that is, without strong left predominance. All or most of the obvious lefthanders probably belong to this group. Thus, Gloning et al. (1969) and Satz, Achenbach, and Fennel (1967) have argued that lefthanders are likely to become aphasic regardless of lesion side and that pure right-sided dominance is unusual. The anomalous language dominance group probably includes many individuals in addition to obvious lefthanders. Luria (1970) found that although almost all patients with penetrating wounds in the primary speech areas on the left became aphasic as a result of their injuries, a year later about 30% had made good or excellent recoveries. Lefthanders and righthanders with left handed first-degree relatives were most likely to be in this group, but they did not constitute the entire good recovery group. We offer the speculation that the 35% without a larger left planum make up this group. Our guess is that this group will include most nonrighthanders (a term we will define more precisely later), as well as most of those with childhood learning disorders and a large proportion of those with first-degree relatives in either of these categories. Gordon (1980) found superior performance on right hemisphere tasks in all members of a group of childhood dyslexics and in nearly all their first-degree relatives. A more recent paper by Gordon (1983) adds further evidence. Much more study will be needed, however, before this can be accepted.

Despite the advances that CT scans have allowed in the study of the brain, there is at least one important limitation on the use of CT scan asymmetries in determining anomalous dominance. The childhood dyslexic whose left hemisphere anomalies were described by Galaburda and Kemper (1979) had a larger temporal lobe on the left. Since the publication of that paper the brains of three more childhood dyslexics have been studied, all of whom have shown similar lesions, predominantly on the left. In all three cases the left temporal lobe was larger than the right. This is probably explained by the presence of neuronal migration defects on the left; that is, the larger size of the left hemisphere was the reflection of abnormality, just as the greater size of the brain in megalencephaly reflects delayed neuronal migration. Some individuals with anomalous dominance, especially those with learning disorders, may thus have an apparently normal pattern of radiological brain asymmetry. If anomalies of this type are common, radiological studies in life may be unreliable indicators of the pattern of lateralization. It is important to realize that imaging techniques are not adequate substitutes for direct anatomical studies. Another problem may relate to the actual ability to predict asymmetries in functionally specific architectonic areas from large-scale CT asymmetries. In a recent study we found no significant correlation between large-scale hemispheric symmetry and asymmetry in a functionally relevant architectonic subdivision of the rat neocortex. Thus, asymmetry in a large portion of brain, such as those measured in CT scans, may not reflect specific functional asymmetries (A. M. Galaburda, personal observations, 1985).

5.3 Asymmetry of Pathways

Flechsig (1876) pointed out an asymmetry in the number of pyramidal fibers crossing from one side to the other in the medullary decussations in about 40% of postmortem human brains. Yakovlev and Rakic (1966) reported asymmetry in the pyramidal decussations of newborn and fetal human brains. In a study of 158 adult brains Kertesz and Geschwind (1971) found that the decussation of the left pyramidal tract occurred more rostrally than that of the right in 82% of cases. Yakovlev and Rakic noted further that a complete decussation was commoner for the pyramid arising from the left hemisphere than for the pyramid arising from the right, which they considered compatible with greater control by the left hemisphere than by the right over the opposite upper limb. Because of the apparently small number of non-righthanders in the study of Kertesz and Geschwind, the pyramidal asymmetry could not be correlated with handedness. The relative lack of nonrighthanders was most likely an artifact, since the handedness information obtained from the surviving relatives was probably unreliable.

Another asymmetry is found in the lower medulla (Smith 1904): an aberrant circumolivary bundle deriving from the pyramidal tract is present on the left side much more commonly than on the right. It is believed by some that the aberrant bundle is destined to innervate the facial nucleus of the opposite side. This asymmetry would thus provide an anatomical substrate for the control of some of the speech-related muscles on the dominant side. The literature also contains data on asymmetries at lower levels of the central nervous system in other species, which we will discuss in chapter 6.

Certain asymmetries in the peripheral nervous system have been well known for many years, for example, those in the sympathetic and parasympathetic systems, which reflect the distribution of autonomic fibers to grossly asymmetrical structures such as the heart, the gut, and the solid abdominal organs. In view of the asymmetries in the intrathoracic and intraabdominal organs, it is likely that there are marked differences in the pattern of visceral sensory innervation from the two sides.

5.4 Cytoarchitectonic Asymmetry

Cytoarchitectonics refer to the characteristic arrangement of neurons in different structures that render them distinguishable from their neighbors. Among the features studied are cell size and packing density, the presence of particular cell types (for instance, pyramids and Meynert stellates), and, as in the case of the cortex, the arrangement of neurons into layers and columns of specific widths and densities. Although gross anatomical features such as gyri and sulci may mirror to a great extent the boundaries of cytoarchitectonic areas, they probably also reflect the actions of physical forces exerted by the brain and skull. Since individual architectonic areas differ in connections and physiology, they are probably functional units (see figure 5.7).

Asymmetries in the volumes of specific architectonic areas have

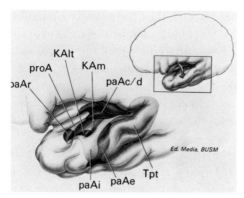

Figure 5.7
Semidiagrammatic rendition of the auditory architectonic divisions on the human
temporal lobe (Galaburda 1984). Area Tpt (temporoparietal) has features common to
the other auditory areas and the association areas lying on the inferior parietal
lobule. Lesions involving this portion of the superior temporal gyrus often result in
disturbances of language function, suggesting that area Tpt comprises an important
element of Wernicke's speech area. Reprinted by permission of Harvard University
Press.

been demonstrated for several regions involved in language function. Thus, area Tpt is usually larger on the left. This area, part of the
extended cortical auditory representation, is located predominantly
on the planum temporale and posterior third of the lateral surface of the superior temporal gyrus (Galaburda and Sanides 1980).
Galaburda et al. (1978) have shown that the magnitude of the asymmetry in Tpt correlates positively with gross asymmetry in the planum temporale; because of its location Tpt is a major contributor to
the asymmetry of the planum. This region makes up a portion of the
classical Wernicke's area, so that Tpt is probably an important part of
the anatomical substrate of language lateralization (see figure 5.8).

Another asymmetrical architectonic area is located in the pars oper-
cularis of the frontal lobe. In eight out of ten brains examined in one
study (Galaburda 1980) this opercular area was larger on the left side,
with six brains showing a volume asymmetry in excess of 30%. The
specific frontal area that is larger on the left is found at the center of a
region lesions of which tend to lead to Broca's aphasia.

The left inferior parietal lobule also participates in language function, but the architectonic parcellation of this region did not receive detailed attention in the past. In a recent study Eidelberg and
Galaburda (1984) parcellated the parietal lobes of nine normal human

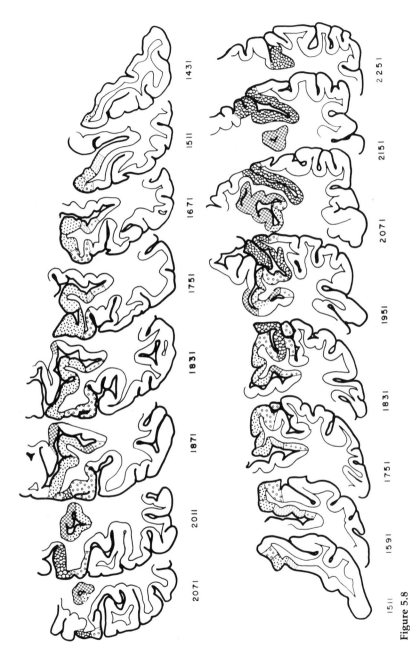

Figure 5.8
Serial sections of the human temporal lobe depicting parcellatons of the auditory architectonic subdivisions. Area Tpt is shown in the cobblestoned pattern; note that it extends both more rostrally (section 1831) and more caudally (section 2251) on the left side (lower series), thus paralleling the longer posterior extension of the left Sylvian fissure.

brains and found asymmetry in cytoarchitectonic area PG, which lies on the angular gyrus. These investigators also found a significant positive correlation between planum asymmetry and asymmetry in the volume of PG. Furthermore, they postulated that size asymmetries in the cortex may be linked so that several areas involved in similar functions will be larger on one side. They suggested that the planum temporale, the inferior frontal gyrus, and the inferior parietal lobule would contain certain areas that are usually all larger on the same side of a given brain. Since the number of cases so far studied is small, the existence of discordant cases cannot be ruled out. In the same study Eidelberg and Galaburda demonstrated asymmetry that favors the right side of another parietal area, PEG, located on the dorsal lip of the inferior parietal lobule. Because of the architectonic and connectional characteristics of area PEG, these authors postulated a role for it in visuospatial function.

Asymmetries in sizes of neurons have also been shown. H. L. Seldon (personal communication) found that Golgi-impregnated neurons were on the average larger in the left than in the right primary auditory cortex. As a result, there were thicker columns and broader intercolumn intervals on the left side in Nissl-stained sections. Dendritic contacts were greater in number in the right auditory association cortex area TA.

Lesion and stimulation data have shown that certain subcortical regions, especially in the posterior thalamus and usually on the left side, are also involved in language function (Luria 1977; Mohr, Watters, and Duncan 1975; Samarel et al. 1976; Graff-Radford et al. 1984). Although the left pulvinar is most often involved in language disorders resulting from thalamic damage, no consistent asymmetry has yet been demonstrated for this nucleus. In eight out of nine brains studied by Eidelberg and Galaburda (1982), however, the lateralis posterior nucleus was larger on the left. This nucleus, part of the posterior thalamic complex, closely abuts the pulvinar and is also likely to be involved in language functions.

5.5 Chemical and Pharmacological Asymmetry

Lateral asymmetries in the content of several transmitter substances and enzymes have been demonstrated in animal and human brains. The most extensive studies are those carried out by Glick and his coworkers in the rat (Glick et al. 1974; Glick and Cox 1978), which have established the existence of chemical and pharmacological asymmetry beyond any doubt. We will deal with this pioneering work in chapter 6; here we will confine ourselves to studies in the human.

Oke et al. (1978) have shown an asymmetry in content of norepinephrine in the human thalamus. The left pulvinar contains more norepinephrine than the right, whereas the ventrobasal complex of the right side is richer in this neurotransmitter than the left. A chemical asymmetry has been reported in the human cerebral cortex as well. Amaducci et al. (1981) showed that the left Brodmann area 22 (part of which corresponds to area Tpt) contained greater cholineacetyltransferase (CAT) activity than the same region on the right. The asymmetry becomes more striking posteriorly in the region of area Tpt. Glick, Ross, and Hough (1982) have found a linked pattern of chemical asymmetries in the human brain.

To our knowledge, the first demonstrations of pharmacological asymmetry in any species were the studies of Szara (1957) and Sai-Halasz, Brunecker, and Szara (1958), who found that dimethyltryptamine, a psychotogenic serotonin derivative, produced both subjective and objective left body findings in human volunteers. Gentili and Tiberi (1963) reported similar findings with diethyltryptamine. Serafetinides (1965) administered LSD-25 (another drug related to serotonin) pre- and postoperatively to 12 patients who underwent right anterior temporal lobe removals and to 11 with left-sided ablations. The typical perceptual responses to LSD disappeared after right, but not left, temporal lobectomy. This finding, which has not to our knowledge been investigated by any other group, might of course have several explanations. One particularly interesting possibility is that lateralized differences in the responses to a drug administered systemically might result from an asymmetrical distribution of receptor sites. Mandell and Knapp (1979) reported asymmetry in serotonin distribution in the rat. Other recent data are also compatible with asymmetrical actions of transmitters in humans. Thus, elementary left-sided neurological signs that disappear after treatment have been reported in depression (Brumback and Staton 1983), and our own experience conforms to these reports (Freeman et al. 1985). Drug-induced dyskinesias have also been reported to occur more often on one side (Waziri 1980), but later studies question this result.

5.6 Development of Asymmetry

Since anatomical asymmetries have been found even during early brain development, they cannot be ascribed exclusively to postnatal influences, although a role for these cannot be excluded. A Sylvian fossa is visible soon after the 10th week of gestation, and a higher right Sylvian point is distinguishable at least by the 16th week (LeMay and Culebras 1972) (see part B of figure 5.3).

Wada, Clarke, and Hamm (1975) were the first to show that the planum asymmetry described in the adult brain is present in the fetus and newborn, and Chi, Dooling, and Gilles (1977) have shown that it can be observed as early as the 31st week of gestation.

Petalias are also seen in the brains of fetuses and children. LeMay (1976) studied photographs of 49 fetal and newborn brains from the Yakovlev collection at the Armed Forces Institute of Pathology (Washington, D.C.) and from the Eunice Kennedy Shriver Center in Waltham, Massachusetts. The left hemisphere was longer in 24, the right was longer in only 8, and they were of equal length in 17. Asymmetries have also been reported in the lengths of the lateral ventricles in brains of children from 5 months to 18 years of age. McRae, Branch, and Milner (1968) reported that in 100 consecutive pneumoencephalograms (87 in righthanded individuals) the left occipital horn was longer in 60%, the right occipital horn was longer in 10%, and the two were symmetrical in 30%. The 75 young patients of Strauss and Fitz (1980) had a longer left occipital horn in 29 cases (39%) and a longer right horn in 13 (17%), with symmetry in 33 cases (44%). If cases with probable damage before the first year of life were excluded, however, the left horn was longer in 54% and the right was longer in 8%, with symmetry in 38%. These data are compatible with the following interpretation. Assume that the probability of unilateral brain damage was equal on the two sides. When the damage was on the left, it would in the majority of cases affect a left occipital horn that was already longer. By contrast, damage on the right would usually increase the size of a horn that was smaller. The net effect would be to produce a proportionally greater increase in right-longer cases.

It was observed early in the nineteenth century that the gyri and sulci often appear at different times in the two sides of the brain. Hervé (1888) called attention to the earlier gross anatomical development of the inferior frontal region of the right side, as compared to the left, and disagreed with other authors who had claimed the reverse without adequate data. Fontes (1944) showed a similar delay in the appearance of cortical markings surrounding the Sylvian fissure of the left side (see figure 5.9). Chi, Dooling, and Gilles (1977) demonstrated that the sulci of the Sylvian region appear later on the left side; in the case of the superior temporal region some of the cortical landmarks on the left trailed those on the right by one to two weeks. Scheibel (1984) has reported that higher-order dendritic branches in the anterior language area develop later on the left than on the right. It thus appears to be the case that regions on the left side that will be larger in the mature brain develop more slowly than the corresponding areas on the right.

An interesting related observation was made by Wada and Davies (1977). They reported that in a series of infant brains approximately the same proportion of males and females had a larger right planum (14% male, 17.7% female). By contrast, in adult specimens there was a much lower proportion of male brains with a larger right planum (6% male, 16% female). The authors suggested that the left planum may enlarge more than the right after birth, especially in males. The right planum may in fact lose cells, thus increasing the asymmetry. An alternative explanation not considered by Wada and Davies is that more males with a larger right planum may die during the early years of life. We will discuss a third alternative in chapter 19.

As noted earlier, Amaducci et al. (1981) found a higher level of cholineacetyltransferase (CAT) in the left superior temporal region of the adult human. A later study from these investigators deals with fetal human brains ranging in gestational age from 20 to 39 weeks (Bracco et al. 1984). The CAT level in the right temporal region was already at its adult level in this period and was higher than that of the left temporal region even in the oldest fetuses. These data suggest that the delay in maturation of this region on the left persists into the postnatal period. This pioneering study also suggests that neurochemical as well as structural asymmetry must be taken into account if one is to understand lateral differences in function. A larger area has a potentially greater capacity than a smaller one, but the full realization of this capacity can be limited by a lack of full neurochemical development. In later chapters we will present further evidence for the earlier development of the human right hemisphere.

The exact developmental mechanism underlying the asymmetrical rate of development of the cortical markings is not known. We believe

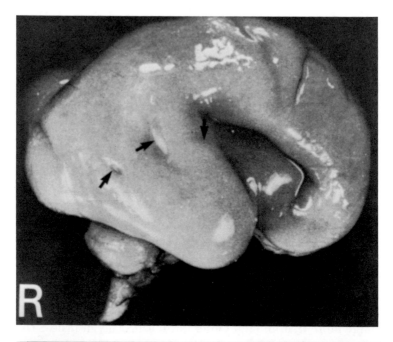

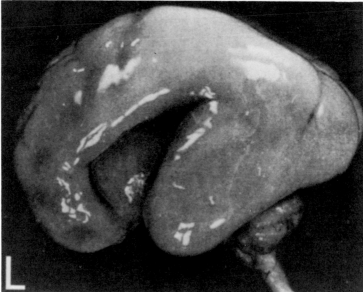

Figure 5.9
Standard asymmetry of the Sylvian fissures in a four-month human fetal brain
showing the upward curve of the right fissure. Also note on the right the presence
of sulci in the temporal lobe and in the supratemporal plane (arrows), which has
been interpreted to denote the more rapid development of these structures in the
right hemisphere.

that asymmetries may date back even to the period of neural induction, when the first primitive neural elements form, and to subsequent early stages of development, so that there may be lateral differences in rates of DNA replication, cell division, neuronal migration, neuropil growth, and cell death. Preliminary evidence from a study performed in the rat suggests that asymmetries in growth rates are present during the period of active neuronal migration. DeBassio, Kemper, and Galaburda (1982) have shown that the stream of neurons migrating to the olfactory bulb of the rat grows at different rates on the two sides, the stream on the right leading the stream on the left. It is interesting to observe that in the rat strain used in these studies the left hemisphere develops more slowly, as appears to be the case in the human. In the rabbit the right optic nerve myelinates in most cases before the left (Narang 1977).

It is important to stress that not every asymmetry in the adult brain is the result of normal development. Some instances of cerebral asymmetry, shown both in postmortem specimens and in radiological studies, may be the result of disorders of hemispheric development. Enlargement of a lateral ventricle, for instance, may reflect an atrophic lesion of the ipsilateral hemisphere. Likewise, reversal of normal petalias seen on CT scans may reflect excessive delays in growth of a hemisphere, most often the left. Unilateral megalencephaly associated with mental retardation has also been described, and the enlarged hemisphere was distinctly the abnormal one (Manz et al. 1979). In the case of childhood dyslexia described by Galaburda and Kemper (1979) the left hemisphere was larger than the right and contained cortex with evidence of abnormal neuronal migration. As we have already noted, one must therefore be wary, especially in clinical populations, of simple interpretations of lateral asymmetries observed by means of radiological methods.

5.7 Evolution of Human Asymmetry

Only a few years ago it was thought that it was impossible to retrace the evolution of human cerebral dominance, since neither the brains of our ancestors nor any records of their linguistic capacities are available. The presence of lateral differences in the Sylvian fissures led LeMay and Culebras (1972) to the unexpected discovery that the asymmetry of brains of ancient humans could be reflected in the impressions on the inner surfaces of their skulls (see part D of figure 5.3).

Several of the gross anatomical asymmetries present in the fetal and mature human brain have been demonstrated in the fossil skulls of our ancestors. The Sylvian fissures often leave their impression on the inner table of the skull. The endocast of the skull of the Neanderthal man of La Chapelle-aux-Saints, who lived 30,000–50,000 years ago, exhibits the typical Sylvian asymmetry of a longer, straighter left fissure and a fissure on the right that turns up at the end. A similar pattern is seen in the endocast of *Sinanthropus pekinensis* (Peking man). The cast of Pithecanthropus I shows a right occipital petalia; the more common left occipital petalia is seen in Pithecanthropus II. Neanderthal skulls often show a left occipital petalia and a right frontal petalia. Holloway and de Lacoste (1982) have shown that skulls of hominoids display the same pattern of asymmetries found in modern humans. Although the skulls of fossil nonhuman primates manifest asymmetry less often than those of humans, when asymmetries are present they show the same patterns as those found in modern humans.

5.8 Right Hemisphere Conservatism

The precocious development of the right hemisphere compared to that of the left deserves some consideration at this point, since it plays a major role in our hypothesis about the influences controlling dominance. Since the right hemisphere develops earlier, those influences during fetal life and early postnatal life acting on the brain are more likely to affect development in the left hemisphere, which is at risk over a longer period. Woo (1931) found greater variability in the left side of the human skull than the right. Since growth of the skull closely reflects brain growth, these data provide further evidence for the greater modifiability of the left hemisphere in development. The earlier development of the right hemisphere is probably not a new phenomenon in humans, but rather one with a long evolutionary history. The development of the individual seems in this regard to recapitulate the course of evolution, a parallel for which there are good reasons in this particular case.

The advantage of earlier development of the right hemisphere derives from its specializations. Among the functions for which the human right hemisphere is dominant are certain types of spatial function, particularly the analysis of external space and the orientation of the body within this space. It also plays a major role in emotion, both in the subjective experience and in the external expression of emotion, as well as in the appreciation of emotion manifested by others. It is also of predominant importance in attention, a not unexpected finding since attentional systems rely heavily on the emotional systems and on spatial orientation. The role of attentional systems in shifting the focus of concentration to external stimuli is of major importance for survival; this is dealt with in detail in the review of Mesulam (1981). The right hemisphere also exerts important controls over certain autonomic activities, as demonstrated for instance by Heilman, Schwartz, and Watson (1977). The right hemisphere thus has a special role in a group of activities essential for survival. It is not surprising that right hemisphere dominance might have appeared early both in the course of evolution and in individual development.

The earlier development of the right hemisphere is probably relevant to what we refer to as the greater "conservatism of right hemispheric function." Although speech and handedness usually depend predominantly on the left hemisphere, there are individuals in whom right hemisphere regions contribute significantly to these functions. There are also those who are especially skillful in use of the left arm, who make up from 6% to 14% of different populations. Aphasia sometimes follows right hemisphere lesions. On the other hand, the appearance, after left-sided lesions, of syndromes typically observed after right posterior hemisphere lesions is less common (for instance, severe persistent right unilateral inattention is uncommon even in lefthanders (Hécaen and Ajuriaguerra 1964)). Furthermore, even lesions of the right hemisphere that lead to aphasia are likely to be accompanied by the typical right hemisphere spatial and emotional alterations.

Since the right hemisphere develops earlier, it is subject to interfering influences over a shorter period of time, and its development is therefore less likely to be impaired. In other words, enlargement of left-sided regions in response to disturbance of the developmental pattern of the right will be less common than the reverse situation, namely, larger size on the right as a result of left-sided delay and subsequent diminished cell death on the right. This probably accounts for the conservatism of the posterior right hemisphere syndromes.

5.9 Mechanisms of Development of Anatomical Asymmetry in the Human Brain

A fundamental question in any discussion of asymmetry is that of its ultimate origins. The system may originally be symmetrical, and some mechanism may later induce asymmetry. An alternative possibility is that asymmetry is present even at the earliest stages—that is, in the ovum itself—as suggested by Corballis and Morgan (1978). It is possible to conceive of mechanisms that could induce asymmetry in a previously symmetrical system, as, for example, in the study of Rogers (1982) on the effect of light on the chick embryo. We will defer discussion of basic mechanisms of asymmetry to chapter 19.

As already pointed out, asymmetry is found in the fetal brain. The photographs of brains of 16-week fetuses in Fontes 1944 reveal the typical asymmetry found in the Sylvian fissures and Sylvian points of the adult. The fundamental pattern of the brain thus appears to be asymmetrical, with the same pattern of asymmetries found in most adults. Metabolic influences on the fetus do not usually alter the direction of this fundamental pattern, which is thus retained by most adults. There are, however, influences in pregnancy that tend to diminish the extent of left-sided predominance, at least in the regions involved in handedness and language, and thus secondarily to result in larger regions on the right side. As noted earlier, our hypothesis is that some factor related to male sex, perhaps testosterone or some closely related factor, is the most likely candidate. The net effect of these intrauterine influences is to produce a shift from left predominance to symmetry, and in a smaller number of cases to modest right predominance.

Several mechanisms could lead to greater relative size on the right. One might speculate that the modifying factor leads to more rapid growth on the right. Conversely, one might speculate that it retards growth on the left. The right side then increases in size because it is more successful in the competition for synapses and therefore undergoes diminished cell death. We believe that the latter mechanism is the correct one; that is, the male-related factor retards growth at least in the language areas of the left side, as evidenced by the impaired neuronal migration and/or assembly on the left side in our cases of developmental dyslexia, which we will describe more fully in chapter 7.

One cannot exclude the possibility that although the most common effect of this factor is to delay growth in the left superior temporal gyrus, it may have other effects in other regions and at other periods in gestation. Migration defects can, of course, be found on the right side, although we suspect, on the basis of evidence to be presented later, that this happens less commonly than on the left. The presence of right-sided migration defects clearly indicates that some influences can cause delayed growth on that side. The predominance of effects in the left superior temporal region may reflect the fact that this area might be at risk over a longer period. It is well known that most teratogens have a "window," a limited period in gestation before and after which they cannot alter some given system. The length of this window may be greater in some regions on the left side. The earlier formation of the right side probably places it at risk over a shorter period. It is likely that there will be variations from individual to individual in the sensitivity of particular regions to the delaying factor. The fact that neuronal migration is slowed preferentially on one side probably implies lateral differences in the chemistry of the system, either in receptor structure or density or even in immune properties, a point to which we will return. It is also possible that there are factors that are operative only at certain periods in development.

The pattern of asymmetry is probably magnified when cell death occurs, since the larger area will be at an advantage in the competition for targets and will attain a more extensive set of bilateral connections. The same influences that delay growth on the left may also slow the growth of axons from cortical regions on the left, thus putting these neurons at a further disadvantage since they may find many targets now occupied by axons from the right side.

Asymmetries in Other Species: Structure, Chemistry, and Function

Since the standard teachings concerning cerebral dominance held that this was a characteristic of humans alone, until the 1960s it was almost universally assumed that functional asymmetry simply did not exist in other species. In tests of handedness individual animals typically showed a consistent preference, but the distribution in the population was evenly divided. In the past twenty years there has been a major revolution in thinking on this matter. Although the work of such authors as Dewson (1979) contained suggestions that functional asymmetry might be found in monkeys tested appropriately, it was Nottebohm and Nottebohm (1976) who clearly demonstrated left cerebral dominance in a nonhuman species, song birds. Another advance came from the work of LeMay and her colleagues (LeMay and Culebras 1972; LeMay and Geschwind 1975), who showed that the anatomical asymmetries found in the Sylvian fissures of the human brain are also present in the brains of great apes. Sherman and his coworkers (1980) demonstrated the presence of functional asymmetry in a mammalian species, the rat.

It is curious, however, that knowledge of anatomical asymmetry in the brains of other species goes back many years. For example, Larrabee (1906) demonstrated early in the century the striking asymmetry of the decussation of the optic chiasm in the trout and the cod, and Kappers, Huber, and Crosby (1936) reported the presence of a consistently much larger right habenular nucleus in the lamprey. It is intriguing to consider why these findings failed to excite the interest of students of human cerebral dominance and why researchers in animal behavior did not explore the possible functional implications. The belief that animals could not possess functional asymmetries and the rejection of anatomical asymmetry as the basis for human dominance probably account for the neglect of these data.

6.1 Asymmetries in Animals

Differences between the hemispheres—anatomical, functional, and chemical—have recently been found in the brains of some nonhuman species. (See table 6.1.) In addition to the asymmetries found by LeMay and Geschwind in the Sylvian fissures of great apes (see part A of figure 5.3), Yeni-Komshian and Benson (1976) have found a larger left planum temporale in the chimpanzee, and Cain and Wada (1979) have documented a larger right frontal lobe in the baboon (see figure 6.1).

Asymmetries in structure have been noted in the brains of cats (Webster and Webster 1975; Kolb et al. 1982), although these are inconsistent. On the other hand, regular anatomical asymmetries have been demonstrated in the rat. Diamond, Johnson, and Ingham (1975) found that the cortex was significantly thicker in several areas on the right than on the left in male rats, whereas in female rats the left-sided areas were thicker. In females ovariectomized at birth the male pattern was seen, which suggested that ovarian hormones modified morphological asymmetries in the female cortex. In a later study Diamond (1984) found that removing the testes in newborn male rats also led to a reversal of the asymmetry pattern in several cortical regions. We have shown as well that the total neocortex, the primary visual area, and the sensorimotor cortex may be larger on the right side in the rat (Sherman and Galaburda 1984). The motor zone is symmetrical, but definitive conclusions must await the examination of additional cases. Asymmetries have been reported in the hippocampus by Diamond et al. (1982, 1983), and we have also found similar lateral differences.

In nonmammalian species several anatomical asymmetries have been reported. Braitenberg and Kemali (1970) reported consistent asymmetries in the size and shape of the habenula in amphibians and fish. Furthermore, Engbretson, Reiner, and Brecha (1981) report that the parietal eye of the lizard, a photosensitive structure, has asymmetrical connections with the habenula (see figure 6.2). The functional significance of these architectonic and connectional asymmetries remains to be studied.

Developmental asymmetry has been found in the rabbit. Narang (1977) described the usually earlier myelination of the right optic nerve as compared with the left, and this correlates with asymmetry

Table 6.1
Anatomical asymmetries in brains of nonhuman species

Structure	N	L>	L=R	R>	Comments
Nonhuman primates					
Skull (Henschen 1926)	6	6	⋯	⋯	Left occipital skull prominence found in old male gorillas
Skull (Groves and Humphrey 1973)	11	4	⋯	1	Difference in length of two sides of skull in gorillas
Sylvian fissure (Cunningham 1892)	⋯	X^1	⋯	⋯	Length of fissure in mangabee chimpanzees
Sylvian fissure (Fischer 1921)	24	50	33	17	Percentage with longer Sylvian fissure; chimpanzees
Sylvian fissure (LeMay and Geschwind 1975)	12	0	2	10	Height of Sylvian point in orangutan
Sylvian fissure (LeMay and Geschwind 1975)	9	1	4	4	Height of Sylvian point in chimpanzee
Sylvian fissure (LeMay and Geschwind 1975)	7	0	5	2	Height of Sylvian point in gorilla
Sylvian fissure group with other Sylvian fissure (Yeni-Komshian and Benson 1976)	25	80	12	8	Percentages with asymmetries in Sylvian fissure length; chimpanzees
Frontal lobe (Cain and Wada 1979)	7	0	1	6	Frontal petalia in baboons

Study	Description				
Temporal lobe (Ingalls 1914)	Difference between posterior ends of Sylvian fissure and superior temporal sulcus in Old World monkeys	...	25	5	30
Other mammals					
Total hemisphere (Kolb et al. 1982)	Weight differences in cat	18	0	7	25
Total hemisphere (Kolb et al. 1982)	Width of hemispheres in cat; percentages	41.1	51.1	7.8	30
Total hemisphere (Kolb et al. 1982)	Height of hemispheres in cat; percentages	47.8	41.1	11.1	30
Total hemisphere (Kolb et al. 1982)	Width of hemispheres in rabbit; percentages	30.8	55.6	13.6	27
Total hemisphere (Kolb et al. 1982)	Height of hemispheres in rabbit; percentages	30.8	55.6	13.6	27
Total hemisphere (Kolb et al. 1982)	Weight of hemispheres in mouse	10	0	4	14
Neocortex (Diamond, Johnson, and Ingham 1975)	Percentages of measures showing asymmetry in cortical thickness; rats and rat pups	94	...	...	225
Neocortex (Diamond, Dowling, and Johnson 1981)	Male rats with thicker cortex in area 17	18	...	...	20
Neocortex (Diamond, Dowling, and Johnson 1981)	Male rats with thicker cortex in area 39	15	...	...	...
Neocortex (Diamond, Dowling, and Johnson 1981)	Female rats with thicker cortex; difference not significant	...	...	8	9
Neocortex (Oswald 1969)	Percentage of male brains with thicker cortex; rats	71	...	...	42

Table 6.1 (continued)

Structure	N	L>	L=R	R>	Comments
Neocortex (Oswald 1969)	54	9	...	...	Percentages of female brains with thicker cortex; rats
Neocortex (Sherman and Galaburda 1982)	11	1	2	8	Volume of neocortex in male rats
Neocortex (Sherman and Galaburda 1982)	9	5	3	1	Volume of neocortex in females; not significant
Neocortical sulci (Webster and Webster 1975)	39	...	55	...	Percentage with symmetrical fissure patterns; in 45% patterns were asymmetrical; cats and kittens
Central region (Kolb et al. 1984)	10	...	...	10	Cross-sectional neocortical area in rats
Hippocampus (Valdes et al. 1981)	18	...	...	...	Mean weight of left hippocampus 64 ± 6 mg; mean weight of right hippocampus 58 ± 11 ($p \leq .001$); rats
Hippocampus (Sherman and Galaburda 1984)	17	1	3	13	Hippocampal volume in handled, environmentally enriched rats; male and female
Hippocampus (Sherman and Galaburda 1984)	15	11	1	3	Hippocampal volume in nonhandled, standard environment rats; female
Hippocampus (Robinson et al. 1985)	24	...	...	14	Weight in male rats; not significant
Hippocampus (Robinson et al. 1985)	23	...	...	14	Weight in female rats; significant
Optic nerve (Narang 1977)	24	5	...	19	Earlier opening of eye in rabbit during postnatal development

X^1: indicates only category where examples were found, although no numbers were provided

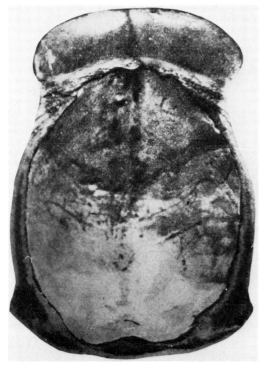

Figure 6.1
Skull of the gorilla John Daniels II. It shows the phenomenon of petalia, or indentation of the inner table of the skull by the underlying brain, involving the left occipital lobe. A similar left occipital petalia has been reported in the human brain. From Clark 1927; reprinted by permission of the *Journal of Anatomy*.

in functional maturation. This study documents once again the precociousness of a right-sided neural structure.

Functional asymmetries have been demonstrated in nonhuman primates, the rat and other rodents, and birds. Peterson et al. (1978) described ear asymmetries for the perception of conspecific calls in Japanese macaques, and Dewson (1979) reported functional asymmetries in auditory discrimination tasks in macaques in studies with temporal lobe lesions.

Asymmetries have been found in rats in open field activity, maze running, and swimming, as well as in tail position. In addition, studies of the effects of lateralized lesions in a variety of rearing conditions have shown that, as in the human, the right hemisphere of the rat subjected to early handling mediates certain aspects of emotional behavior (Denenberg 1981).

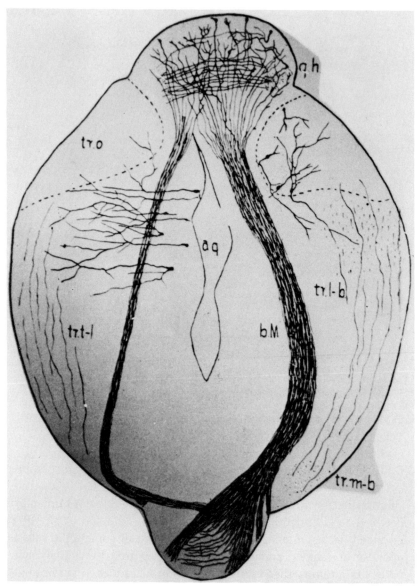

Figure 6.2
The habenular nucleus of several fishes, amphibians, and reptiles is strikingly asymmetrical. This diagram shows an asymmetry of the habenulopeduncular tract in petromyzons, illustrating that some asymmetries of cellular structures have known associated asymmetries in patterns of connections. From Johnston 1902; reprinted by permission of the *Journal of Comparative Neurology*.

In nonmammalian species the most striking demonstrations of lateralization of function are those of Nottebohm (1980) in singing birds. In finches and canaries song is abolished by lesions of the left side of the brain but not by lesions of the right side. Nottebohm has shown striking size differences in the song control nuclei between singing male and nonsinging female birds but has failed to reveal right-left anatomical asymmetries. Asymmetries in visual discrimination and auditory inhibition have also been demonstrated in chicks (Rogers 1980).

Chemical and pharmacological asymmetries can also be demonstrated in animals. In the last several years research in normal rats has established asymmetries in striatal dopamine content (Zimmerberg, Glick, and Jerussi 1974), striatal dopamine receptors (Schneider, Murphy, and Coons 1982), striatal dopamine metabolism and dopamine-stimulated adenyl cyclase activity (Jerussi and Glick 1976; Robinson, Becker, and Ramirez 1980), striatal deoxyglucose uptake (Glick et al. 1979), and striatal GABA turnover (Starr and Kilpatrick 1981). These biochemical asymmetries have been correlated with the preferred direction of rotation after administration of amphetamines and the direction of spontaneous nocturnal circling. Additional asymmetries have been demonstrated in nucleus accumbens, thalamus, hippocampus, neocortex, and other structures. In several of these studies sex differences in asymmetry of structure and function have been found.

6.2 Implications of Animal Asymmetries

The demonstrations of asymmetry in animals appear to confirm the belief that biologically determined asymmetry has existed throughout vertebrate evolution and that human asymmetries are neither a recent development nor an example of convergent evolution but rather only the most recent example of a fundamental feature of neuroanatomy and behavior.

Biological, psychological, and medical research always sustains an important impetus from animal models, which permit experimental manipulations that cannot be carried out in humans. Data from such models have led repeatedly to revisions of theories based only on studies in normal humans and those with brain lesions.

It should be possible to breed experimental strains for marked asymmetry of specific structures, or for marked functional asymmetry, and thus to carry out studies on highly uniform animals, in contrast to the necessarily high variability of human groups. This method should also render possible experimental study of different mechanisms of asymmetry, and in particular of the effects of manipulations during pregnancy and early postnatal life. It will also be easy to study the effects of pregnancy during different seasons and under differing conditions of light, temperature, and other variables.

Experimental animal studies may be particularly useful for investigation of functions that have long been thought to be confined to the human, such as language. The common response that such study is not possible in view of the lack of convincing evidence of language function in any other species is, we believe, based on a narrow view of language. Human language depends on specific brain regions, which must have evolved, and which probably share common activities with homologous areas in other species.

In the recent heated discussions about whether apes could acquire language the implications of asymmetries found in the chimpanzee brain in areas homologous to the language regions of humans were completely neglected. If destruction of such a homologous cortical area on the left side had abolished the asserted linguistic capacities of the animal, this would have supported the belief that it had learned some activity related to human language. If on the other hand the animal's acquired abilities had been abolished only by bilateral ablations of nonhomologous regions, the argument against the possession of linguistic capacities would have been supported.

One of the major stumbling blocks to a study of language forerunners in other species is the assumption that language is primarily a means of communication between humans. This has led investigators to stress the training of animals to *produce* language. Yet humans clearly use language as an internal processing mechanism. The fact that this is usually perceived as inner speech has strengthened the assumption that this must reflect the internal use of learned language. The interconnected language areas must, however, possess a method of neural coding. We suggest that such internal codes exist in other species and are used for internal cognitive processing. The external communicative aspect of language may have been a late development in the human, but the fundamental features of an internal language system may have existed at a far earlier period.

If such systems are present in lower species, investigators may be guided to them by the presence of anatomical asymmetries similar to those found in the human. It should be possible to breed animals for increased size of these regions. One could also use the technique devised by Goldman (1978), that is, placement of lesions during fetal life in one area, so as to increase the size of the corresponding contralateral area or of adjacent areas. The development of animals with superior functions of these regions might permit cognitive studies that could illuminate as yet unexpected features of language. Such studies should be guided by information concerning the possible homologues of human language regions, for example, the above-mentioned asymmetries in the planum temporale of the chimpanzee and the Sylvian fissures of the great apes.

Similarly, the lack of animal models has delayed the study of psychiatric illnesses. The described relationships of some of these to handedness suggest that dominance plays an important role. As the study of lateralized brain disorders in psychosis advances, it should be possible to carry out studies on the functions of homologous unilaterally asymmetrical regions in other species. Data from such models will perhaps make it possible to restate the concept of psychosis in new—and perhaps unexpected—terms that are more susceptible to neurological and cognitive analysis than those now available.

The study of animal models has already revealed some intriguing findings: the poorer maze performance of rats who do not show strong turning tendencies to either side (Zimmerberg, Strumpf, and Glick 1978), the importance of early experience in establishing dominance in male rats (Sherman et al. 1980), altered callosal projection patterns in animals with early visual system lesions (Innocenti 1981; Cynader, Lepore, and Guillemot 1981), and the higher rate of left-turning in females who have been in utero with many males (Glick 1983). Animal studies have already cast important light on mechanisms of asymmetry in the claws of crustaceans (Mellon 1981; Govind and Kent 1982) and in the chick brain (Rogers 1982). Since animal models will probably be available in very large numbers, the possibilities for important additions to and modifications of ideas concerning dominance are almost without limit.

7   Pathology of Asymmetry in Developmental Learning Disorders

Just as asymmetries in the structure of the hemispheres may begin to appear at least as early as the period of neuronal migration, so changes in the pattern of cerebral lateralization may result from factors operating at different stages of the normal developmental process. Gross alterations of symmetrical structures have been produced experimentally. The formation of paired optic vesicles may be altered by a lesion during the time of neural induction (Alderman 1935). Damage to the chordal plate portion of the mesoderm at that period produces an amphibian embryo with a single midline eye. Kallen (1967) has suggested that drugs such as thalidomide might act at this early stage by producing errors in the induction of ectodermal structures in the limbs. As we will note later, many influences that lead to abnormal limb formation act primarily on one side.

Evidence from the study of brains of individuals with developmental dyslexia (a specific disorder of language in the face of normal intelligence) suggests another mechanism, occurring later in fetal development, which may lead to disorders of lateralization. Because of its relevance to our hypothesis, we will consider this evidence in some detail.

7.1 Neuropathology of Developmental Dyslexia

Neuropathological findings in the brain in developmental dyslexia have been described in three cases, and preliminary observations are available in two more. In the first case Drake (1968) reported excessive numbers of neurons in the subcortical white matter, especially in the parietal region, which suggested a disorder of neuronal migration. He did not, however, mention any significant lateral differences.

Anomalies were also found at other levels; for example, an arteriovenous malformation was found in the cerebellum.

A second case, reported by Galaburda and Kemper (1979), was studied with particular attention to lateralization of abnormalities and to cytoarchitectonic structure. The findings in that case may be summarized as follows: (1) a large area of micropolygyria (a malformation of cortex consisting of abnormal folding, fewer layers, and primitive orientation of neurons, thought to result from an alteration in neuronal migration) in the left planum temporale and posterior third of the superior temporal gyrus, (2) clusters of neurons in layer one of the cortex (see figure 7.1), especially in the superior temporal gyrus, and (3) abnormal, primitive layering and primitive neurons in numerous perisylvian and pericingulate areas. These abnormalities were present only in some parts of the left cortex, and none were found on the right. Later review disclosed five small ectopias involving right frontal cortex.

The findings in a third case included primitive left hemisphere cortical differentiation and frank cortical dysplasias, especially in perisylvian cortex, and clusters of ectopic neurons in layer one, some associated with brain wart formation (see figure 7.2). In this case again the right hemisphere cortex was more normal (Galaburda 1983).

Preliminary findings in a fourth case have included bilateral cortical dysplasias and ectopias in the temporal lobes, both more striking on the left side. A fifth case, recently studied, has revealed similar findings (Galaburda et al. 1985).

Additional architectonic abnormalities in the thalamus of the Galaburda and Kemper case have been reported by Galaburda and Eidelberg (1982). The medial geniculate nucleus and the lateralis posterior nucleus were distorted in shape and showed clusters of primitive cells and abnormal myelination. In contrast to the abnormalities in the cortex, those found in the thalamus were more symmetrical. This brain was also abnormal on gross examination. The left hemisphere was large and contained an excessive volume of subcortical white matter. Asymmetrical enlargement of a single hemisphere has been reported in a case of unilateral megalencephaly (Manz et al. 1979), which involved the right hemisphere of a 13-month-old infant with intractable seizures. The cortex was simple in gyral pattern and abnormal in cytoarchitecture, with clusters of primitive neurons and indistinct cortical layering. The subcortex contained cells arrested in migration.

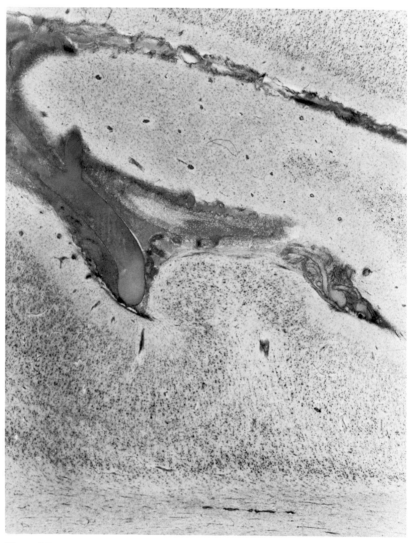

Figure 7.1
Photomicrograph of a representative cortical ectopia taken from the left temporal lobe of the brain of a dyslexic man. The extrusion of ectopic neurons distorting the pial edge has caused this form of anomaly to be dubbed "brain wart." This and related brain abnormalities are thought to originate during mid pregnancy and have been postulated to reflect injury during this developmental period. More extensive brain disorganization may underlie these types of focal defect.

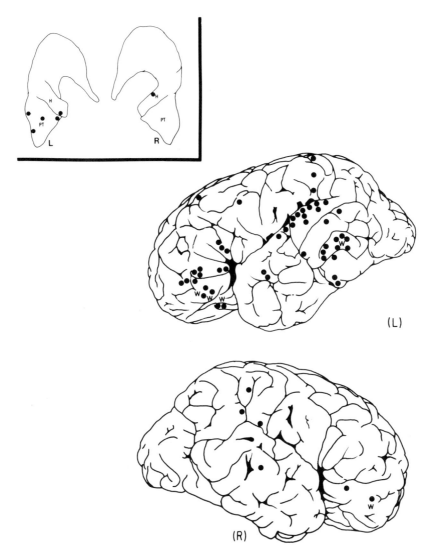

Figure 7.2
Diagram of the cerebral hemispheres and planum temporale (inset) from the brain of
the dyslexic of figure 7.1. Note that the planum temporale exhibits the symmetrical
pattern, as it does in all cases studied to date. The closed circles on the drawings of
the cerebral convexities depict areas of ectopia and related cortical anomalies. Note
that the involvement is strikingly asymmetrical. W, brain wart.

It has often been noted that malformed cortex frequently contains abnormal blood vessels. Arteriovenous malformations (AVMs), which are more common in males than females, are often found in the posterior perisylvian regions. Levine, Hier, and Calvanio (1981) have reported a case of learning disability in a young patient who had undergone a left temporal lobectomy following a hemorrhage probably originating in an AVM. They suggested that the developmental reading disorder in this case was the result of the acquired lesion. It is quite possible, however, that the AVM was embedded in abnormally developed temporal cortex, so that the patient would probably have been dyslexic even if the malformation had not ruptured. We are aware of six patients with lifelong reading disability but no early history of bleeding or surgery, who were shown to have AVMs in the left temporoparietal region (see figure 7.3). Caron et al. (1982) reported a series of AVMs in the language areas of the left hemisphere. The population was overwhelmingly male, and although left superior temporal AVMs were common in the men, none were found in the women. Persistent aphasia occurred infrequently after surgery, suggesting that speech representation was anomalous in most of these cases. In another series from Japan (Mori et al. 1980) cortical AVMs were found predominantly in males on the left side.

In summary, the brain abnormalities in dyslexia are developmental in nature and can be attributed to alterations in the cortex and connectionally related subcortical structures resulting from disturbances in neuronal migration and assembly. It is likely that in some individuals the postulated slowing of the rate of migration of neurons to the left cortex is even more marked than in the normal state; this excessive delay can lead to lateralized developmental arrest and malformation, thus leading to childhood dyslexia and possibly other developmental disorders.

It is conceivable, furthermore, that delay of left cortical development results in more successful competition by right hemisphere neurons for available synapses and thus leads to diminished rates of neuronal death on the right. This would explain the reported excess of reversed asymmetries in severe dyslexics (Hier et al. 1978; Hier, LeMay, and Rosenberger 1979; Rosenberger and Hier 1980); but these have not yet been confirmed. We wish to stress again that in the four dyslexics studied at postmortem in our laboratory we have found not reversal of the usual asymmetry, but symmetry of the planum temporale. The potential for enhanced right hemisphere development in the

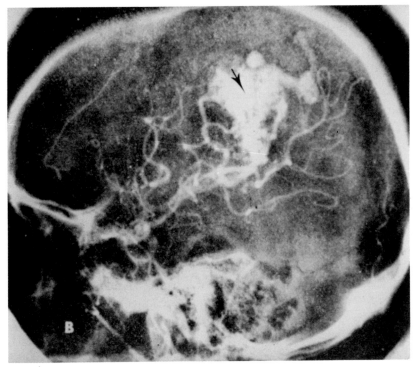

Figure 7.3
Lateral view of an arteriogram showing the branches of the left internal carotid artery. The radioopaque blush (arrow) in the temporoparietal region represents an arteriovenous anomaly. Such anomalies are developmental in origin, and this radiograph was obtained in an adult patient with life-long developmental dyslexia. Also see text.

dyslexics helps to explain the apparent excess of lefthandedness and right hemisphere skills in dyslexics and their families (Gordon 1980, 1983).

7.2 Are Minor Neuronal Migration Defects Normal?

Neurologists and neuropathologists have usually regarded extensive disorders of neuronal migration and assembly as dramatic abnormalities typically associated with mental defect and epilepsy, whereas the pathological significance of less severe and more localized malformations of this kind has in general been neglected. It has often been tacitly assumed that although gross disorders produced rather crude neurological defects, those of lesser degree are of little significance (with one important exception, namely, that minor migrational defects are accepted as causes of epilepsy).

The common ascription of little importance to minor developmental defects is based on the belief that they are frequently found in normal brains. This standard teaching may, however, be erroneous. The assertion that these defects are not associated with neurological impairment means only that they are found relatively frequently in the brains of patients who have died of nonneurological illness and in whose records no mention is made of neurological disorder. It is, however, clear that a wide variety of neurological defects without relatively crude manifestations are overlooked by most physicians. Despite the high frequency of the many forms of learning disability, they are rarely mentioned in medical records, even on neurological services, and histories of mental illness are often not sought after. Patients and families often fail to mention these conditions either because they do not regard them as medical illnesses or because they wish to conceal them. If facts about learning disability or psychiatric disorder are not obtained from the patients themselves, the errors in family histories are even greater. It is extremely rare to find a reference to dyslexia in a sibling or to stuttering in an uncle. Furthermore, good personal histories of handedness are rarely obtained, even on neurological services, and are almost never recorded in other departments; familial histories of handedness are almost entirely lacking. Even when such data are obtained, they are usually of low reliability.

The fact that we couple allusion to the failure to obtain histories of learning disabilities, handedness, and psychiatric disorders with a discussion of the tendency to dismiss lesser degrees of anomalies of neural development as of little or no pathological significance is deliberate. We suspect that precisely this type of "minor" developmental pathology is responsible for many of the learning disabilities and related disorders and psychiatric conditions. Support for this hypothesis comes from the study of Veith and Schwindt (1976), who found a much higher rate of minor anomalies in autopsy brains of social derelicts than in those of other individuals.

Another form of developmental anomaly that is probably even more widely overlooked than minor migrational disorders is failure of normal maturation of neuronal organization within a particular brain region. Neuropathologists who usually deal with adult material do not always have experience with developmental patterns and may thus overlook failures of full maturation of neuronal assemblies. A disagreement about the postmortem findings in a case of Tourette syndrome illustrates this problem. Balthasar (1957) concluded that the caudate nucleus of his patient with Tourette syndrome showed a cytoarchitectonic pattern usually seen only in infancy. Eminent students of the pathology of the basal ganglia disagreed about the validity of these conclusions.

These problems illustrate some standard conceptions concerning the teratology of the nervous system. Many congenital malformations such as neural tube defects are correctly regarded as causes of gross neurological disorder, but the possibility that apparently minor degrees of these conditions may have important effects on function receives much less attention. In agenesis of the corpus callosum the entire structure or major portions of it are absent. It is unlikely that the underlying causes of this condition will manifest themselves only in such gross deficits; there are probably many individuals in whom certain portions of the corpus callosum contain a much smaller than normal complement of fibers. Recent studies (Goldman 1978; Innocenti 1981; Cynader, Lepore, and Guillemot 1981) confirm that the local pattern of callosal connections can be altered by intrauterine or postnatal interventions and thus make it likely that such cases exist. Such a condition should be reflected in accompanying functional changes, although of a different and less coarse nature than those seen in patients with total agenesis. The same may be true of neural tube defects.

7.3 The "Pathology of Superiority"

There is another possible, although surprising, reason why lesser degrees of neuronal migration deficits or of other forms of teratology may be overlooked. We have already suggested that in mild cases of this type certain kinds of disturbed function may commonly occur. We must consider another apparently paradoxical possibility: that minor malformations may often be associated, not with abnormal function, but with distinctly superior capacities in certain areas. The idea that a "pathological" disorder could manifest itself primarily by superior abilities is alien to standard modes of thinking about neurological disease. It may seem bizarre to speak of "the neuropathology of superior intellectual functions"; yet we suggest that a superior outcome, with or without accompanying problems in other areas, is not at all unusual. The reasons have already been advanced. If the growth of one portion of the hemisphere is delayed, then other regions will be larger than they normally would have been. When this increase in size is marked, superior or even remarkable talents may develop.

A likely example of such reciprocal increased development is afforded by the patient reported by Galaburda and Kemper (1979) who despite lifelong difficulties in reading was a talented metalsmith. The superior right hemisphere talents of dyslexics documented by Gordon (1983) illustrate the same point. The patient reported by Sano (1918) manifested remarkable artistic talents in the face of very limited linguistic capacities. On the basis of careful comparison with control cerebra, Sano concluded that the brain of this individual showed poor development in both frontal and temporal lobes but markedly enlarged posterior regions. The remarkable talents of some autistic patients (Rimland 1964, 1978) possibly represent further examples of the operation of this mechanism.

The occurrence of high talents through this mechanism may also help to explain the high frequency of such disorders as childhood dyslexia. The high spatial talents of many of the affected individuals may counteract the evolutionary disadvantage of their disabilities. This would, of course, be even more conspicuously the case in nonliterate societies, in which failure to learn to read would not be a problem. Even in a literate society the manifest disability may be overcome through great effort and good teaching, so that only the superior talents may be evident. The fact that family members may manifest the high talents without obvious disabilities raises the possibility that serious difficulties may occur in only a fraction of those in whom left hemisphere development is slowed to a greater degree than in most people. These considerations raise the possibility that the mechanisms that delay left hemisphere growth have been selected in the course of evolution because they often produce individuals of elevated talent. The advantage of these individuals presumably outweighs the disadvantage of the learning disabilities, which probably appear in a small number in whom the slowing on the left is excessive. Again, a disability such as dyslexia would have been of minor importance in nonliterate societies.

8   Standard and Anomalous Dominance

Individual patterns of brain dominance have important biological associations, such as increased susceptibility to certain disorders and a higher likelihood of possessing certain talents. Classifying individuals according to dominance patterns is difficult, however, and the simple twofold classification into right- and lefthandedness presents many problems that have not received the attention they deserve. In this chapter we will discuss some of the differences in dominance patterns. Since the literature is vast, we will emphasize issues relevant to our hypothesis.

8.1 Anomalous Dominance: Definition

Although differences in manual preference were probably recognized in early human societies, it was not until Broca's discovery of cerebral dominance for language that it was appreciated that handedness reflected some aspects of brain organization. Many of the early concepts have, however, turned out either to be incorrect or to distort the true situation.

The discovery that lesions producing aphasia lay predominantly on the left led to the belief in a *single* dominant hemisphere that controlled both handedness and speech. It is now clear that one can no longer speak of a dominant and a nondominant hemisphere, since each side of the brain is dominant for certain functions. It is also appropriate to discuss briefly the belief that handedness and language dominance are closely linked.

It may appear at first that this question can be answered by statistical means: are righthandedness and left hemisphere speech associated more often than would be expected by chance? The problem is complex, however, since there are continuously distributed degrees of language lateralization and handedness. Even if one neglected this and accepted the common view that strong righthandedness is more often associated with left language dominance than strong lefthandedness, this would only mean that dominance for handedness and dominance for speech were not *statistically* independent; it would not answer the basic biological question. An example should illustrate this.

Assume that two species of plant are always found in the same geographical locations; that is, their ranges are strongly associated statistically. The association might be obligatory; each species might depend on the other for some essential substance. At the other extreme, it might be possible to show experimentally that one species could be grown independently of the other. Their common geographical ranges would then simply reflect some common mode of spread or common requirements for certain types of climate and soil.

In the same manner the nonrandom association of handedness and language dominance might or might not reflect a deeper physiological connection. Consider the fact that both the heart and the spleen are almost always located on the left side. The existence of cases in which the heart is located on the right but the spleen lies on the left suggests that there is no obligatory link between the sites of the two organs.

Applying these considerations to handedness and speech one might entertain the possibility that they were intrinsically linked. On the one hand, they might both be manifestations of the same neural substrate, or the development in the embryo of the substrate for one might inevitably cause the substrate of the other to develop on the same side. On the other hand, they might have independent neural substrates.

The assumption that handedness and speech are intrinsically linked runs into many difficulties. There are occasional strong righthanders who become aphasic after right hemisphere lesions. Furthermore, although a higher percentage of lefthanders than righthanders become aphasic after right hemisphere lesions, the majority of permanent severe aphasias in lefthanders are the result of left hemisphere damage (Goodglass and Quadfasel 1954). Despite these findings, the fact that the great majority of righthanders become aphasic after left hemisphere lesions has kept alive the idea that speech and handedness are intrinsically linked.

Our thinking has been influenced strongly by the ideas of Annett

(1978a,b) on random dominance. She postulates the existence of people in whom dominance for handedness and language may be random, that is, in whom either hemisphere may be dominant for either function. We make the assumption that language and handedness depend on separate neural substrates that do not necessarily develop at the same periods. It is likely, however, that the basic brain pattern in most humans is one in which the left hemisphere contains the separate brain regions involved in language acquisition and in the learning of certain types of motor skills. The neurological substrates of these functions probably develop according to different schedules. Certain prenatal retarding influences might be operative to a marked degree during the development of either, or both, of these functions. If the degree of retardation is sufficiently great, the initial anatomical advantage in the left hemisphere will be diminished and the two sides will exhibit a greater degree of symmetry. The more nearly symmetry is achieved in some particular region, the more likely there will be random dominance for the function subserved by that region. In the majority of people both functions will remain left hemisphere dominant, but there will be a majority in whom either, or both, will be randomly determined or occasionally clearly shifted to the right. If either can be shifted independently of the other, it is likely that there is no strong intrinsic linkage.

It should be clear that our hypothesis regarding the cause of random dominance differs in some respects from Annett's. She believes that in about 18% of the population dominance is random and that in these people accidental factors determine the lateralization of language or handedness. The remainder of the population carries a "right-shift" gene that increases the probability of left hemisphere dominance for these functions. By contrast, we postulate that in most humans there is an innate bias toward left hemisphere dominance for both of these functions and that certain influences during fetal life act to diminish this innate bias and thus to create random dominance. Like Corballis and Morgan (1978), we believe in a "left-shift" factor. This factor is influenced by genetic endowment, but there are large nongenetic components. (It should be noted that Annett has stressed the importance of nongenetic factors in the determination of dominance patterns. We do not wish to overemphasize the differences between our interpretation and that of Annett, whose innovative ideas on random dominance have so profoundly influenced our thinking.)

The majority of the population and, of course, an even larger majority of righthanders exhibit the *standard dominance pattern:* strong left hemisphere dominance for language and handedness, and strong right hemisphere dominance for other functions. Even in this group the degree of dominance of any given function will vary somewhat from person to person.

The term *anomalous dominance* refers to those in whom the pattern differs from the standard form. There is no sharp cutoff point at which one can speak of a shift from standard to anomalous dominance. Our rough estimate is that anomalous dominance will be found in approximately 30% to 35% of individuals, roughly the percentage in whom the planum temporale is not larger on the left side.

It is important to stress anomalous dominance rather than lefthandedness. According to Annett's formulation, lefthanders comprise about half of those in whom handedness is random. She estimates that random handedness is present in 18% of the population, of whom about half, or 9%, will be lefthanded. Our tentative formulation differs from Annett's in one respect. She postulates that the same 18% have random dominance for language. We speculate that about 30% of the population will have random dominance (with occasional clear shifts to the right hemisphere) for language or handedness, and sometimes, but not always, for both. We believe that random dominance for language may be more frequent than random dominance for handedness, although this remains to be confirmed experimentally. Our basis for this view is again speculative, namely, that the as yet unknown neural substrate for handedness may develop earlier and over a shorter period than that for language. For this reason the shift from left hemisphere to random (or reversed) dominance for handedness will be present in fewer individuals than a similar shift for language functions. Thus, many people in whom language dominance is random will also have random handedness, but the postulated later development of the speech regions will make possible random language dominance despite a standard pattern of dominance for handedness.

There is another, much less speculative argument in favor of our belief that individuals need not have random dominance for all functions. As noted in section 5.8, certain aspects of right hemisphere dominance are very conservative; that is, they are rarely shifted to the left hemisphere even in individuals with anomalous dominance for language and handedness. In our view, the rarity of anomalous dominance of right hemisphere functions reflects the earlier and more rapid development of that side of the brain, which is thus less subject to modulating influences.

In the anomalous dominance group there will be various degrees of deviance from the more uniform pattern of the larger group with standard dominance. Because the anomalous dominance group will consist of people in whom the development of asymmetry has been altered at different periods and to different extents, they will be a more variable population and will have to be considered on a more individual basis.

Annett's concept that in some cases laterality is randomly determined may appear to be daring but, as she herself points out, there is a well-documented example. In hereditary situs inversus (transposition of the viscera) in mice (Layton 1976) only half of the offspring of a mating of parents homozygous for the disorder will have reverse situs. Yet the apparently normal offspring have themselves as high a percentage of affected offspring as do their abnormal littermates. The gene thus appears to determine not reverse situs but rather random situs. Another possibly related example is afforded by Kartagener syndrome (Afzelius et al. 1978), in which one finds repeated bronchial infections associated with situs inversus. There are, however, children with apparently similar disorders of the cilia of the respiratory tract who lack reversed placement of the viscera. Dahlberg (1944–47) also called attention to genes whose unilateral manifestations may appear on either side.

There have been several attempts to distinguish subpopulations among lefthanders. Some studies stress the distinction between *familial lefthanders* (those with lefthandedness in close relatives) and *nonfamilial lefthanders*. Although we believe that this distinction may be important, we will refer to it only occasionally. Another distinction is commonly made between *normal* and *pathological* lefthanders. There are, of course, some individuals who have sustained either in utero or in early childhood a considerable degree of damage to the left hemisphere and who therefore necessarily end up having right hemisphere dominance for language and handedness. Although the term "pathological lefthandedness" is appropriately applied to this group, we agree with Annett that this concept has probably been too widely applied. It should be obvious from the discussions in this book that many lefthanders who do have visible abnormalities in the brain— such as the childhood dyslexics discussed earlier—have had their brain organization altered by an extreme case of the same mechanism that produces the majority of normal lefthanders. If this hypothesis is correct, then the frequent equation in the literature of "genetic" with "normal" lefthandedness and of "acquired" with "pathological" lefthandedness must be erroneous. We do not accept the equating of *normal* with *genetic* lefthandedness, since, as we will show, the intrauterine influences producing lefthandedness are only in part genetically determined. Furthermore, those genetic influences that favor the development of lefthandedness will also favor, in a small proportion of cases, the development of the anomalies of neuronal migration that lead to dyslexia. We would not subscribe to the view that our hypothesis is equivalent to that of Bakan (1971, 1977), that all lefthandedness is pathological. The essential point is that there is a continuum between the cases of lefthandedness with and without accompanying disorders.

We have suggested that a major cause of anomalous dominance is markedly delayed development of a left hemisphere that is initially programmed for strong left-sided dominance for speech and handedness. The effect of the delay is primarily to create individuals who have more symmetrical brains, although a few will be reversed. A second, uncommon cause of anomalous dominance is early extensive damage to the left hemisphere. A third possibility should be considered as well. It is conceivable—and, we believe, entirely possible—that individuals exist who are endowed with a right hemisphere that is in fact the mirror image of the left hemisphere of the majority of the population—that is, individuals who have true "cerebral situs inversus." We will discuss this issue in chapter 19.

8.2 The Assessment of Handedness

The assessment of handedness deserves comment. Benton, Meyers, and Polder (1962) have stressed that self-described lefthanders are a highly variable group. Other investigators, however, argue that it is unnecessary to carry out elaborate measurements of manual preference because there is a high agreement between handedness as measured by test and self-described handedness. It is easy to see why the high correlation between self-described handedness and test scores is of little use. Even if the correlation were high—say, 0.8—this would mean, according to accepted standards, that 64% of the variance would be accounted for. This means that a considerable fraction of the variable would be unexplained and that there would be many discrepancies, most of which would be present in exactly those individuals of greatest interest—those with anomalous dominance.

There is a close parallel between this situation and the relationship between speech and handedness. In a very high percentage of cases the side of an aphasia-producing lesion can be predicted if the handedness of the affected individual is known. It is precisely the small number of discrepant cases that are the object of interest.

In our own population studies we have used the Oldfield Handedness Battery (1971), although in later studies we have modified both the items and the scoring. Although we have postulated that deviations from righthandedness might identify only about one-third of the anomalous dominance group, lefthandedness is still a very valuable marker, because it is readily measurable. For many reasons, only some of which we will discuss, it is probably the case that, despite their usefulness, existing tests of handedness have serious shortcomings and that better tests incorporating recent conceptual advances should be developed.

The Wada test (Wada and Rasmussen 1960) deserves comment in this regard. It is often assumed that this test, the intracarotid injection of sodium amytal frequently used to determine dominance for language, is an unequivocal test of unilateral or bilateral speech representation. If this assumption is accepted, it might be concluded, for example, from the data of Rasmussen and Milner (1977) that lefthandedness was more common than anomalous language representation. Of the 214 nonrighthanded epileptics studied by Rasmussen and Milner 50% had left hemisphere speech by the Wada test and the remaining 50% had bilateral, or right-sided, speech. As the authors themselves point out, this population of epileptics cannot be necessarily regarded as typical of the general lefthanded population. There is, however, another point to make about the interpretation of the Wada test, namely, that it underestimates the proportion who have significant degrees of bilateral language representation. Luria (1970) reported that aphasia was present in the acute stage in nearly all soldiers with penetrating brain wounds in the primary speech areas in the left hemisphere. A year after their injuries the rate of recovery from these left-sided lesions was much higher among lefthanders and among righthanders with familial lefthandedness. It might be assumed that all of these individuals (had they been tested before their injuries) would have become aphasic after injection of amytal into the left internal carotid, but the test would have given no clue about which ones would recover from such a lesion, since regression of aphasia in those who improved often took weeks or months. In brief, the Wada test can demonstrate right hemisphere participation in language but it cannot exclude it, since the right hemisphere linguistic capacity may become manifest only a considerable time after left-sided damage.

We hope that increasingly more accurate markers of anomalous dominance will be developed. In our view, the following individuals are more likely to have anomalous language dominance: (1) lefthanders, (2) righthanders with first-degree lefthanded relatives, (3) righthanders with developmental learning disorders, (4) righthanders with first-degree relatives with learning disorders. In support of criteria 1 and 2 is Luria's (1970) finding that individuals in these groups had a higher rate of recovery from aphasia. By neuropsychological testing, Gordon (1980, 1983) has found evidence for anomalous dominance in both dyslexics and their relatives. One implication of this classification is that members of groups 3 and 4 should also have higher rates of recovery from aphasia. Preliminary observations suggest that this may be the case, but an extensive study will be necessary.

There are other reasons why measurements of handedness have been problematic. Exclusive reliance on the hand used for writing presents many difficulties. As pointed out by Gloning et al. (1969) in a study done about thirty years ago, all of their Austrian lefthanders had been compelled to write with the right hand in school, and even today this practice is the rule in many countries. The greater tolerance shown toward lefthanded writing in the English-speaking countries might lead to the assumption that in these communities the writing hand could appropriately be used as a measure of laterality. Yet even in these countries many pressures, both explicit and implicit, favor righthanded writing; this is reflected in the fact that this activity is the most righthanded of all.

Another source of difficulty is the common assumption that there are two separate populations: righthanders and lefthanders. Unfortunately, the criteria for separating the two groups vary from test to test. Even altering some of the items on a test may alter the individual's classification, as was shown by Provins, Milner, and Kerr (1982).

Furthermore, Annett (1970) has stressed that handedness, like height, is a continuous variable. In studying the associations of handedness, the appropriate question is therefore not, "Is lefthandedness more common in condition A than in the general population?" but rather, "Is the distribution of handedness scores different in condition A from that in the general population?" A recent example shows the value of this approach. In a study of 99 alcoholics (Nasrallah, Keelor, and McCalley-Whitters 1983) the proportion who were frankly lefthanded was the same as among the 86 controls (about 7.0% with the test used in this study). The proportion of alcoholics and controls who were not frankly righthanded differed widely, however: 56% as compared with 30%, respectively, a highly significant result.

Another problem stems from the inclusion in some "handedness" batteries of items relating to eye dominance, such as, "Which eye do you use in looking through a microscope?" This actually may weaken the data since, as has often been shown (Porac and Coren 1981), replies on eye-dominance questions correlate poorly with items on hand usage. As we will soon show, even the use of pure motor dominance items may present difficulties.

A recent study of over 1,000 professionals illuminates several of these points (Schachter and Galaburda, in press). A modified form of the Oldfield Handedness Battery was employed. Instead of setting arbitrary cutoffs for lefthandedness, the numbers of individuals in each range of laterality scores were counted, adjacent cells being pooled only to meet the requirements of the chi square test. A history of dyslexia was found in 9% to 10% of those with scores in the ranges from −100 (complete lefthandedness on this test) through +70 and then dropped sharply to about 3% in the ranges above this level. Thus, the data showed that +70 was a cutoff point. Of the dyslexics 56% scored +70 or lower as compared with 22% of the nondyslexics. By contrast, 20% of the dyslexics wrote with the left hand as compared with 10% of the nondyslexics. Thirty percent of the dyslexics but only 15% of the nondyslexics were self-described lefthanders or ambidexters. The data from this study show that the writing hand and self-described handedness are much less sensitive measures than consideration of the entire distribution of laterality scores.

8.3 Other Aspects of Motor Dominance

Since the concept of handedness has played so great a role in all considerations of dominance, some potentially important distinctions

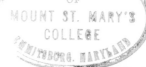

deserve further discussion. The very term "handedness" has had an important impact on the directions of research on motor dominance. Manual preference can be assessed relatively easily either by questionnaire or by tests of performance. Adroit use of the hand is a cardinal biological feature of humans and underlies many skilled activities. Many laterality questionnaires consist primarily of questions about activities carried out with one hand, such as writing or using a spoon. Liepmann (1908) proposed that handedness was a reflection of the greater capacity of one side of the brain to acquire the programs for particular motor skills. Righthandedness would thus imply that an individual's left hemisphere was more capable of learning how to carry out certain unimanual skilled movements. We accept this formulation and therefore believe that the lefthander is someone whose right hemisphere is superior at acquiring these programs. More generally, the nonrighthander is someone in whom the right hemisphere has some significant capacity for acquiring at least certain motor programs. It should be noted that some investigators would not agree with this formulation, since they believe that even in some lefthanders the left hemisphere may be superior at acquiring motor programs (Kimura and Archibald 1974).

In contrast to the stress on unimanual skill, there has been much less emphasis on other forms of motor dominance, although one can find data on preferences for using one leg or foot. We do not consider so-called eye dominance, since it is not clear that it reflects any type of *motor* dominance. However, we believe there is another form of motor learning that may also depend primarily on one hemisphere, although it is not immediately evident to the observer, namely, the learning of activities that depend to a considerable extent on coordinated movements of the trunk and the limbs.

Someone who could not learn to hold a pencil or a fork properly might be described as clumsy. This term might also be applied to someone who could not readily acquire the coordinations necessary for riding a bicycle, dancing, or pole-vaulting. Since the latter type of skill is not *obviously* lateralized, it has not entered into studies of cerebral dominance. Since muscles of both sides of the trunk are used in these activities in coordination with limbs on both sides, it may seem odd to postulate dominance for them. Even if they were controlled predominantly from one hemisphere, it would be difficult to determine the leading half of the brain by either questionnaires or tests of performance. That activities dependent on bilateral innerva-

tion might be controlled by one side of the brain should not be surprising. With rare exceptions, the sounds of language are produced
by symmetrically innervated muscles and yet are typically programmed unilaterally. Furthermore, in singing the same muscles are
innervated bilaterally and yet may be controlled from the side of the
brain contralateral to the one controlling speech. In fact, the movements of both speech and singing are far more symmetrical than
many movements involving the trunk. It is commonly pointed out by
coaches that ice-skaters find it easier to execute turns in one direction
than in the other.

Some people, such as those with high athletic or dancing talents,
are superior in acquiring these truncal skills. Others, such as painters
of miniatures or those who carry out delicate dissections, are particularly adept at learning activities that require high degrees of manual
adroitness. It is a common, although unfortunate, practice to characterize skills involving the trunk as gross and those involving the hand
as fine. There is no reason to presume that the skill of the great ballet
dancer is less refined than that of the neurophysiologist who places
an electrode inside a cell. Everyday observation is consistent with the
possibility that the two forms of skill can be independent. Accounts of
childhood dyslexics often exemplify this contrast. The first patient
studied by Galaburda and Kemper (1979), described as clumsy in gait
all through development, became a skilled metalsmith. Another typical case known to us is a female dyslexic described as clumsy and
unathletic—that is, deficient in the handling of the trunk—who is a
highly skilled painter of miniatures.

Although there may be several ways to account for these discrepancies, one possible explanation is that there may be more than one
form of motor learning. One type might be described as *pyramidal:* the
ability to learn programs of complex sequences of separate joint
movements, especially in the fingers. (For reasons that need not be
discussed, the term "contralateral pyramidal" might be more appropriate, but the shorter term will be used here.) Another form of motor
learning might be described as *axial:* the ability to acquire programs of
movements of the trunk and eyes along with coordinated limb movements. The axial system is also commonly involved in control of
proximal movements at the limb girdles. This distinction has been
discussed in an analysis of the apraxias (Geschwind 1975). The two
types of movements have on the whole quite separate representa-
tions in the brain. Complex sequences of finger positions depend

primarily on purely contralateral motor systems arising in the pre-
central gyrus, whereas axial movements depend on several other
cortical areas, the outflow from which is distributed bilaterally. The
programs for axial learning, like almost all other complex cognitive
functions, probably depend primarily on one hemisphere. It is therefore reasonable to hypothesize that these two forms of motor dominance are independent and that the degree of intrinsic talent can be
different in each system.

   We believe that in those with standard dominance the programs for
both types of motor dominance lie in the left hemisphere but that
under conditions of anomalous dominance they may lie in separate
hemispheres. Evidence to support this view is at present only fragmentary. Gesell and Ames (1947) described the tendency of newborn
infants placed on the back to turn the head and trunk to one side. Of
the children studied, 90% were righthanded at age 10; all of these had
turned to the right at birth. The 5% who at birth had turned to the left
were all lefthanded at age 10. There remained, however, 5% who had
turned to the right at birth but were lefthanded at age 10. One speculative possibility is that in this group axial and pyramidal dominance
were located in different hemispheres.

   There are other fragmentary but suggestive observations. We have
now found many individuals who use the left hand to write on paper
but the right hand to write at the blackboard or to paint. Ordinary
writing requires many separate finger movements, but painting and
writing at the blackboard require few, if any, finger movements and
control is exercised predominantly at the shoulder girdle. Further
observations are consistent with this hypothesis. One woman uses
the left hand for writing and sculpting but the right for painting. The
German artist Menzel painted with the right hand but did engraving
with the left hand, which he also used for writing (Keller 1942). Another person known to us writes on paper with the right hand, but in
charcoal drawing produces outlines of figures with the left hand and
then fills in details with the right.

   These observations are compatible with the possibility that there
are independent forms of motor dominance. Lateral discrepancies in
the hemispheric localization of the two forms of motor dominance
would be most common in the anomalous dominance population. An
implication of this hypothesis is that people in whom different activities are carried out on the left and the right will display a tendency to
clustering; they will preferentially use one hand for pyramidal tasks
and the other arm for axial tasks. Studies are underway to test these

hypotheses and to apply them to laterality testing. If the data are compatible with this hypothesis, certain conclusions would probably follow. It would be easy to understand why laterality batteries with different items might give different results in some people. Furthermore, it is possible that some individuals who are thought of now as having "mixed" dominance may, in fact, have rather pure pyramidal dominance of one hemisphere and equally pure axial dominance of the other. This is not to imply that there will not be other people who may have truly mixed dominance; for example, each hemisphere might possess a significant capacity for learning pyramidal or axial movement programs.

Annett proposes that lefthanders will tend to come from a group with random dominance for handedness. This raises the possibility that in the random dominance group pyramidal dominance will not, on the average, be as strongly localized in one hemisphere as in most righthanders. This possibility gains support from Kilshaw and Annett's (1983) finding that in actual tests of skill lefthanders show, on the average, smaller differences in performance between the two hands than righthanders. This accounts for the fact that many nonrighthanders show a high rate of ambidexterity. Futhermore, such a bilateral representation would lead to a higher rate of overall skill in cases such as bimanual tasks where each hand could make a significant contribution. We suspect that nonrighthanders will also show, on the average, a higher rate of bilateral representation of axial control. The less strongly lateralized pattern of motor skill would help to account in part for the elevated rate of nonrighthandedness among athletes, in contrast to the common view that this is entirely the result of an advantage in competing against righthanded opponents.

8.4 Lefthandedness and Congenital Lesions

We have suggested that lefthandedness is the result in many cases of influences that slow left hemisphere development. Taylor (1975a,b) has presented data that appear to conflict with this interpretation. The cause of temporal lobe epilepsy is in some cases "alien tissue," that is, various types of cell rests, such as the neuronal migration disorders discussed earlier. There is a high frequency of lefthandedness in these cases even when the alien tissue is found on the right side.

Left-sided operations for alien tissue were carried out on 10 males (4 lefthanded (LH)) and 10 females (3 LH); right-sided operations were carried out on 27 males (6 LH) and 9 females (1 LH). By contrast, in the mesial temporal sclerosis group left-sided operations were performed on 16 males (2 LH) and 5 females (1 LH), and right-sided operations were performed on 10 males (2 LH) and 10 females (none LH). Mesial temporal sclerosis is now generally regarded as a lesion acquired in early childhood, probably as a sequel of febrile convulsions. (The fact that the majority of operated cases with alien tissue had right-sided foci cannot be used as a measure of the total frequency of such anomalies in all temporal lobe epileptics, since the operative selection criteria favored right-sided cases. As we will show later, large population studies show an excess of left hemisphere epileptic foci.)

Taylor pointed out that males with alien tissue appear to have an elevated rate of lefthandedness regardless of the side of the lesion and therefore that one could not accept the simple assumption that only those with left hemisphere developmental anomalies would manifest an excess of lefthandedness. These data are, however, not necessarily incompatible with our hypothesis. They are generally in accord with the proposal that lefthandedness is determined by events in utero, since the alien tissue group had a higher rate of lefthandedness than the mesial temporal sclerosis group. Since the right hemisphere develops more rapidly than the left, those with right hemisphere hamartomas are likely to have suffered developmental delays early in pregnancy. The hamartomas found were predominantly in the uncal region, which develops much earlier than the superior temporal lobe. It is possible that in many of these individuals the delaying influences were still active at later stages and might thus retard the growth of later developing left-sided cortical regions and thus favor random dominance. Furthermore, the standard operation, especially on the left, was removal of the temporal lobe anterior to the speech regions. Alien tissue in the superior temporal gyrus, as seen in our dyslexic patients, would not have been found by the pathologist. The type of lesion seen in our dyslexics would not in general be visible on the surface of the brain. The uncal lesion might thus have no effect on handedness or language lateralization but might only be a marker of a disturbing influence in development. Future data concerning patients with alien tissue will be required before their high rates of lefthandedness can be explained definitively. In particular, to our knowledge, there are no data concerning the rates of learning disorders in this population.

9   Associations of Anomalous Dominance

Even today an accumulated body of folklore and prejudices concerning lefthandedness continues to exist. In many cultures powerful taboos persist regarding use of the left hand for certain activities such as eating. In the United States, where tolerance of lefthandedness is perhaps at its highest, a few people still try to inhibit the use of the left hand by children. Because of this body of inherited myths and prejudices, most scientifically trained persons are understandably skeptical concerning asserted behavioral or bodily characteristics of lefthanders. We will not review the many nonscientific beliefs. On the other hand, it has become increasingly clear that individual differences in cerebral dominance reflect variations in brain organization. Furthermore, anomalous patterns of cerebral dominance have many associations, both favorable (such as certain superior talents) and unfavorable (such as particular developmental learning disorders and immune diseases). In this chapter we will discuss some of these variations, which constitute an important body of facts that any adequate theory must account for.

Before describing some of these associations, we must warn against certain misconceptions that could arise concerning our discussion. Some readers might draw the conclusion that individuals with anomalous dominance, and in particular obvious lefthanders, are at a disadvantage in terms of health because of elevated frequencies of certain medical conditions, and at a disadvantage intellectually and psychologically because of higher rates of developmental disorders such as autism, dyslexia, and stuttering.

This conclusion would be erroneous. The fact that one group has a higher rate of certain diseases than another does not mean that it is at an *overall* disadvantage for disability or death. An entire field of medicine and many textbooks are devoted to diseases that occur ex-

clusively or overwhelmingly in women and are important causes of
morbidity and mortality. Yet females have lower death rates than
males at every age. Despite their elevated rates of many conditions,
women have lower rates of other disorders, in particular cardiovascular diseases and certain cancers, which more than counterbalance the
risk of diseases such as ovarian carcinoma.

A study of patients with celiac disease (Swinson et al. 1983) affords
an example of at least a partial balance between risks and advantages.
Patients with this condition exhibit not only a markedly higher frequency of malignant lymphomas and some uncommon gastrointestinal cancers but also a reduced number of lung and breast cancers. In
this case there is a net disadvantage since the total prevalence of all
malignancies is elevated.

In the past emphasis was usually placed on disadvantages of lefthandedness. This grew out of older prejudices that lefthanders were
deviant, and out of beliefs that much lefthandedness was the result of
brain damage. We believe that a full investigation of the disease associations of lefthandedness (and more generally of anomalous dominance) will demonstrate elevated rates of certain conditions but low
rates of others. In particular, we suspect that most infections and
many forms of cancer will be less often found in lefthanders than in
righthanders, but this remains to be studied. Seltzer and Sherwin
(1983) have reported that although lefthandedness is present in elevated frequency in presenile Alzheimer's disease, it is rare in senile
dementia, a far more common disorder. The high frequency of lefthandedness in many populations suggests that lefthanders are not at
an overall disadvantage. Thus, they may have a different pattern of
disorders, but there is no reason to believe that they are less healthy.

A similar argument applies to intellectual and other psychological
features in the anomalous dominance population. One cannot con-
clude that this population is disadvantaged, without surveying the
entire array of psychological attributes. There is increasing evidence
that even in the learning disabled certain talents occur in high frequency. An elevated rate of lefthandedness is found among architects
(Peterson and Lansky 1974) and among the mathematically gifted
(Kolata 1983). There is no reason to assume that either the righthanded or the lefthanded group is superior; it is likely that each
group has a higher rate of certain talents and disabilities than the
other.

It should also be kept in mind that in different societies, or in different stages of the history of one society, the advantages of the two groups may vary in relation to health or accomplishment. Several examples in other areas illustrate this point. When malaria is common, a population carrying the sickle-cell gene will have a high degree of protection, but in the absence of malaria it will be at a net disadvantage. Individuals with high serum immunoglobulin E (IgE) may be at an advantage when parasitic diseases, to which they are probably more resistant, are common (Marsh, Meyers, and Bias 1981), but at a disadvantage, because of their high rate of asthma, when these diseases are rare. Great physical strength was once an advantage in nearly all societies but now is of little importance in technologically advanced communities, whereas mathematical talent, of minor importance in the past, is in great demand. Dyslexia is of little importance in nonliterate societies. It is quite possible that the overall relative advantages of those with anomalous and standard dominance are different in different societies and at different epochs.

A common misconception is reflected in comments we have frequently heard: "I know many exceptions to these findings," "There are lots of healthy lefthanders," and so on. It is, of course, clear that most people with anomalous dominance do not suffer from the conditions mentioned and that what is being described are higher relative rates of certain conditions.

9.1 Learning Disabilities and Anomalous Dominance

The term "developmental learning disorders" is applied rather loosely to a group of conditions with onset before puberty, characterized by difficulties in acquisition of speech or certain cognitive functions or in anomalies of emotional development. It includes both some disorders recognized by the ancients, such as stuttering, and others recognized only in the recent past, such as developmental dyslexia. The current list includes developmental dyslexia (which is probably the most common), stuttering, delayed speech, childhood autism, and hyperactivity. Although Tourette syndrome is usually not listed, it has many of the same features. This list is almost certainly incomplete, and there are probably many other conditions with delimited behavioral difficulties. Thus, Weintraub and Mesulam (1983) have recently described a group in which disorders of social adjustment predominate, but we will not include this in our discussion, since much more information needs to be collected.

These conditions have certain common properties, one of which is a preponderance of males; the greater tendency of females affected with some of these conditions, such as stuttering, to improve with age leads to a further increase in the male majority. The available genetic studies reveal a rather similar pattern of inheritance. Affected individuals are more likely to have affected relatives than normal controls. The minority of affected females tend to have more affected relatives and more affected children than the males. These conditions appear to be interrelated; for example, if one identical twin is autistic, the other twin, when not autistic, is more likely to have one of the other learning disabilities (Folstein and Rutter 1977). Orton (1925) commented on the increased rate of stuttering among dyslexics, and Ludlow et al. (1982) found a similar relationship between Tourette syndrome and dyslexia.

Another common factor is an elevated frequency of personal and familial nonrighthandedness, as noted by Orton in his very first descriptions of dyslexia and as found in many later studies. Porac and Coren (1981) point out that although some studies deny an increase in lefthandedness in the dyslexic population, no study has ever found the reverse, namely, a deficiency of lefthandedness.

The study of Geschwind and Behan (1982) lends strong support to the existence of this association. In most earlier investigations patients with some form of learning disorder were assessed for handedness. In our study groups were instead chosen for handedness and then assessed for personal and familial histories of learning disorders. In this initial study we compared only individuals with laterality quotients of -100 (very strongly lefthanded persons) and $+100$ (very strongly righthanded persons). Two separate studies gave very similar results. The pooled figures of the two studies show that 11.8% of the 500 strong lefthanders reported learning disorders, compared to only 1.1% of the 900 strong righthanders. In both series there was also a significantly higher frequency of learning disorders among the first- and second-degree relatives of the lefthanders than among those of the righthanders. A third series has yielded similar results (Geschwind and Behan 1984). The rate of dyslexia was fifteen times as high in the strong lefthanders as in the strong righthanders, and stuttering was five times as common in the lefthanders.

The more recent study discussed earlier, based on a group of over 1,000 professionals who completed a modified form of the Oldfield Handedness Battery, provides further data on the association of dyslexia and handedness (see Schachter and Galaburda, in press). With the scoring method used (slightly modified from the original), a score of greater than +70 was attained by about 75% of the respondents. In order to attain a score above +70, there can be either at most one item out of ten for which the respondent reports predominant use of the left hand or at most five items for which the respondent reports occasional use of the left hand. Dyslexia was reported by 3% of those scoring above +70. In both the ranges from 0 to +70 (about 15% of the population) and 0 to −100 (about 10%) the rate of dyslexia was 9%. The probability of this distribution was less than 0.001. In other words, even a minor degree of deviation from full righthandedness was associated with a sharp rise in the frequency of dyslexia. Yet many of the individuals in the 0 to +70 range described themselves as righthanded, and most wrote with the right hand. This illustrates the point discussed earlier that it is important to ascertain whether the distribution of laterality scores in those with a given condition is different from that in the general population. In some cases there may be a marked shift to the lefthanded end, but in others, when the shift is of lesser degree, it may be demonstrated only by a significant decrease in the proportion of those at the righthanded end and an increase in those in the middle ranges.

It should also be noted that these findings do not imply that non-righthandedness is the cause of the learning disorder; we regard non-righthandedness only as a marker of an alteration in dominance. Nor do these findings imply that one should expect the majority of individuals with learning disorders to be nonrighthanded, although this may turn out to be true in some instances.

We cannot deal here in detail with the reasons for the many disagreements in the literature. Again, our initial investigations in Glasglow used a method different from that used by others, in that we studied individuals at the extremes of the handedness scale. Moreover, the study reported by Schachter and Galaburda (in press) was confined to professionals, most of whom had completed graduate studies, whereas most investigations have been carried out with children. Although in our studies the individuals identified themselves as dyslexics, it is difficult to see how such huge differences could have resulted from a concealed selection bias.

The published data on autism and stuttering show less disagreement than those on reading difficulty. Autistic children have a far higher rate of nonrighthandedness than normal controls (Boucher

1977; Colby and Parkinson 1977). Bishop (1983) reports five studies on stammerers or stutterers, all showing a higher rate of nonright-handedness than controls; in three the differences are very large. Obviously, stuttering is diagnosed with less uncertainty than reading disorder.

These data are compatible with the hypothesis that the influences that favor nonrighthandedness will in extreme cases lead to an increased frequency of learning disorders. In future research it will be important to study the brains of patients with conditions other than childhood dyslexia, such as autism and stuttering, and especially the brains of frank righthanders and of females who suffered from these conditions.

The onset or worsening of many conditions at or near puberty strongly suggests a major role for sex hormones. Temporal lobe epilepsy resulting from alien tissue commonly starts at this time, and neurofibromatosis and scoliosis worsen. Of interest are the behavioral conditions (such as anorexia nervosa, which primarily affects females), which appear predominantly after puberty. The rarer puberty onset male condition, Kleine-Levin syndrome (Oswald 1969), is in many ways the opposite of anorexia nervosa, both in sex distribution and in clinical features. Kleine-Levin patients have periodic attacks in which they overeat, sleep excessively, and may be sexually hyperactive; all these contrast with the behavior of anorexia nervosa patients, who eat little, are very active, and are typically hyposexual. A recent postmortem report of a case of Kleine-Levin syndrome describes anomalies of formation of certain thalamic nuclei, thought to be of possible viral origin (Carpenter, Yassa, and Ochs 1982). This raises the possibility that some puberty onset syndromes might also be the result of even earlier defects of neuronal migration or assembly. There are still no handedness data for these conditions.

By contrast, other conditions, both neurological and nonneurological, may improve at puberty; this is true of some cases of Tourette syndrome. Other important changes take place at puberty; for example, the average superiority of males in certain aspects of spatial function does not become fully manifest until this age (Vandenberg and Kuse 1979). M. Denckla (personal communication) has commented on the improvement in certain motor functions in many male dyslexics at puberty.

There are other developmental learning disorders that have re-

ceived little attention, despite their frequency and theoretical importance, presumably because they rarely come to medical or educational
attention. Extreme lack of musical ability is one of these; lack of
artistic ability is another. Since most people are relatively poor at artistic activities, it might be worthwhile to conduct studies in the reverse manner, that is, to investigate the handedness and sex distribution of artistically talented children. It would be important from the
point of view of any theory to identify conditions that are predominant in females before puberty and especially those that are more
common among righthanders than among lefthanders.

It is important to point out that one handedness group might contain an elevated proportion both of those with high talent and of
those with distinctly inferior capacities for some particular function. A
hypothetical example might be that of mathematical talent. Recent
studies have supported the view that superior mathematical talents
are more frequent among males (Benbow and Stanley 1983) who have
an elevated rate of lefthandedness (Kolata 1983). It has therefore been
argued by some that special difficulty in mathematics will be more
common in females. This need not necessarily be the case. It is thus
conceivable that males, and even lefthanded males, might be found
more frequently at both ends of the scale. Only further experimental
studies will make it possible to work out the intricacies of some of
these relationships.

The genetic pattern of learning disorders is compatible with the
thesis presented here. The pattern of inheritance has generally been
considered to be compatible with autosomal dominant transmission.
It might appear at first that this conflicts with male predominance. In
genetics a distinction is made between *sex-limited* and *sex-linked* inheritance. An example of the former is male pattern baldness, inherited
as an autosomal dominant (Carter 1972), which is not expressed in
young women because of low levels of dihydrotestosterone. In sex-
limited inheritance a gene is expressed less often in one sex. We have
proposed that learning disorders are more common in males because
of some male-related factor in development, possibly testosterone.
Inheritance will play a role; for instance, genes might affect testosterone levels, sensitivity to testosterone, or a large number of other
factors. As noted earlier, affected females are likely to have more
affected relatives and more affected children than affected males.
According to the hypothesis, a female would be more likely to suffer

from a learning disorder if she were subjected to high testosterone effect during development. This would be especially likely if she had inherited high sensitivity to testosterone.

Although fewer females stutter, they have, on the average, more affected relatives, and they are more likely to have affected children than males who stutter (Kidd, Heimbuch, and Records 1981). It is easy to conceive of reasons for this pattern. If, for example, there were large differences in genetically transmitted sensitivity to testosterone, then females who stuttered would frequently have inherited high sensitivity, since in most cases females would not have exposure to very high levels of testosterone. Many of these females' relatives—and, in particular, many of their children—would share this high sensitivity. On the other hand, males with, on the average, higher levels of testosterone would not require as high a level of sensitivity to testosterone to be subjected to an excessive delaying effect. In particular, the female relatives of a male who stuttered, but did not have high testosterone sensitivity, would be expected to have low rates of the disability. Furthermore, since testosterone levels in male fetuses are sensitive to environmental effects (to be discussed in chapter 11), males could be affected more frequently by environmental causes. There are, of course, other possible explanations for the genetic findings; the above example only serves to illustrate that the greater frequency of learning disorders in males need not imply that affected males will have more affected relatives than affected females.

It should be pointed out that the affected female may have a higher number of affected children for other reasons. The children might inherit a higher genetic sensitivity to testosterone. In addition, certain animal experiments show that exposing females to high testosterone during development is likely to permanently alter their metalbolism (Edwards 1964; Bronson and Desjardins 1968). The child of such a female is thus possibly more likely to be exposed to high androgen levels and therefore to be affected.

9.2 Immune Disorders

The elevated frequency of immune disorders in lefthandedness is also compatible with our theory, since evidence to be given later shows that testosterone affects the development of the immune system.

We use the term *immune disorder* to mean atopic disorders (the allergies, typically of childhood onset), autoimmune disorders, and other conditions in whose pathogenesis immunity plays a major role. There are, of course, certain infections in which the manifestations during the acute stage depend to a major degree on immune mechanisms. Here we will discuss only chronic conditions in which immunity plays a major role, but we will return to the question of infection in chapter 16.

Because of the clinical observation made by one of us (NG) that certain diseases appeared to be more common in lefthanded subjects, a study was carried out in order to investigate these associations (Geschwind and Behan 1982). In our first group of investigations we compared only individuals who on the Oldfield Handedness Battery scored either -100 (complete lefthandedness) or $+100$ (complete righthandedness). The data concerning the increased frequency of learning disorders in the strongly lefthanded subjects have already been given. In the first series 27 of the 253 strong lefthanders reported personal histories of immune disorders, as compared with 10 of the 253 strong righthanders ($p < 0.005$). In the second series the diagnosis of immune disorders was accepted only if it had been made in a teaching hospital. A smaller absolute number of cases were therefore found, but the relative frequencies in the lefthanded and righthanded subjects were comparable to those found in the first study. In each of the studies immune disorders thus occurred about 2½ times as frequently in the strong lefthanders as in the strong righthanders. The lefthanded subjects also reported a higher rate of immune disorders in first- and second-degree relatives. A third study (Geschwind and Behan 1984) has yielded similar results.

Having confirmed the hypothesis that immune disorders occurred more frequently in the strong lefthanded than in the strong righthanded groups, we investigated the reverse association: the frequency of nonrighthandness in different disease groups. Although many different immune disorders were reported by our respondents, we were particularly struck by the apparently high frequency of conditions affecting the gastrointestinal tract (ulcerative colitis, regional ileitis, and celiac disease) and the thyroid gland (for instance, Hashimoto's thyroiditis). The respondents in our first study did not include a large number of cases with these immune disorders, although small numbers of other groups were available. In subsequent studies (Geschwind and Behan 1984) we have found that among patients in Scotland with the gut-associated and thyroid immune disorders, the rates of personal and familial lefthandedness are markedly increased. The same was true for migraine, myasthenia gravis, and atopic diseases such as asthma. On the other hand, we again found no difference from the general population in the rates of lefthand-edness in rheumatoid arthritis. It should be noted that in these studies of particular diseases we used an arbitrary cutoff score of zero as the upper limit of lefthandedness. In future studies the procedure should, however, be the one suggested earlier: instead of assigning arbitrary cutoff points, the logical procedure is to compare the distribution of laterality scores in the patient groups and in the controls. We suspect that, when this method is used, it will be found that some of the other immune disorders will also display significant shifts of the laterality distributions to the left. The method of using zero as an arbitrary cutoff point would, of course, fail to reveal a marked reduction in extreme righthanded scores with a correspondingly marked rise in the range of scores between zero and $+70$.

9.2.1 Design of Future Studies

On reviewing the studies, it is now clear that many details and interrelationships must be worked out. In studying disease groups, one should employ the strategy just outlined of avoiding arbitrary cutoff points. We expect that the degree of shift to the left will vary with different disorders. The use of a cutoff at zero or below will miss disorders in which the shift is less marked but still substantial, a point we will discuss again in other connections.

Experimental design should take other factors into account as well. First, it will be important to study males and females separately. Second, Dr. Marcel Kinsbourne, whose work we will mention in more detail further on, has suggested that important information may be obtained by looking at interrelationships. Thus, will the rate of immune disorder be the same in those with, say, a laterality quotient of -100 who are dyslexic and those with the same score who are not? Furthermore, will dyslexics with strongly *positive* laterality scores have higher rates of immune disorder than nondyslexic individuals with the same scores? Third, it will be particularly interesting to study conditions such as rheumatoid spondylitis (Marie-Strumpell disease), Reiter syndrome, and enteropathic arthritis, all male predominant and all with strong associations with HLA B-27 (histocompatibility antigen B-27).

9.2.2 Implications of the Data

The data presented are compatible with the hypothesis that the factors that influence laterality also affect the development of the immune system and thus lead to a later elevated frequency of immune disorders. An elevated rate of immune disorders was found in strongly lefthanded individuals who would, by hypothesis, have been subject to a greater male-related effect than the strongly righthanded group. It would be important to determine whether there is a "dose effect"—in other words, whether the frequency of immune disorders increases with the degree of lefthandedness.

More light is thrown on these findings by a recent study of M. Kinsbourne and B. Bemporad (personal communication), who investigated a group in a school for children with learning disorders. The rate of immune disorders was significantly higher among families of lefthanded dyslexics than among families of righthanded dyslexics without familial lefthandedness.

Another confirmation comes from a study by Wood (1983), who reported that lefthandedness was more common in patients with autoimmune diseases of the thyroid and in their first-degree relatives than in those with nonimmune thyroid disorders (such as nodular goiter).

In Benbow and Stanley's (1983) study of a large, strongly male-predominant group of mathematically gifted children, the subjects had not only twice as high a rate of lefthandedness as a less gifted group but also five times as high a rate of allergies.

The inclusion of migraine raises several questions. There is some support for the participation of immune mechanisms in at least some cases, for instance, a reported increase in the rate of migraine in lupus erythematosus. During attacks there is an asymmetrical distribution of mast cells (Thonnard-Neumann 1969). In a recent report (Egger et al. 1983) of a controlled study of treatment of childhood migraine with exclusion diets, the authors argue for an allergic mechanism. There are, of course, causes of food intolerance other than allergy. Further studies will be needed to confirm the existence of an immune mechanism in migraine.

Our data also show an increased rate of lefthandedness among those with atopic disorders such as asthma, eczema, and hay fever. It is of interest that atopic disorders usually begin before puberty and are more common in males (Crawford and Beldham 1976), whereas other common immune disorders typically begin after puberty and are more frequent in females. This is in accord with the hypothesis that the postpubertal male, despite a possibly greater propensity toward autoimmunity, is protected from it by his own hormones, whereas this masking effect is weaker before puberty.

The types of immune disorders found most frequently in anomalous dominance populations will be determined more accurately only after more extensive studies. It is worthwhile, however, to speculate briefly on the current findings. According to our hypothesis, the increased tendency to immune disorders is the result of suppression of development of the thymus and other immune organs. It is likely that the delaying effects on brain growth will not be uniform throughout pregnancy and that the particular dominance pattern of any individual will be determined by the exact timing and intensity of these effects. One would expect that the pattern of immune disorders would also reflect the timing of the delaying effects in relation to processes of development in the thymus and other organs. One might guess that at any given time the processing within the thymus of lymphocytes that recognize self would be closely coordinated with the organ systems developing at that time, since the characteristic antigens of those systems will not have been present earlier. The high rate of gut and thyroid immune disorders may give important hints about the usual timing of the disturbing influences in brain development, although other factors, including genetic endowment, may determine special susceptibility of certain systems. In any case we do not wish to imply that a general susceptibility to all forms of immune disorders will exist in all those with anomalous dominance. In fact, the possibility exists that particular forms of anomalous dominance will be associated with particular conditions, although the data available at present are at best only suggestive. The literature on stuttering repeatedly refers to allergies (Diehl 1958; Szondi 1932); pediatric neurologists have repeatedly told us of the high frequency of migraine in dyslexics; Coleman (1976) discusses the high rate of a gut-related disorder in autism.

As a corollary of these findings one might expect that some related conditions, such as lymphoid malignancies that have a close relationship to immune disorder, would also be elevated in the anomalous dominance population. On the other hand, more common forms of cancer might well be less frequent in this group.

Other hypotheses concerning the relationship between immune disorders and lefthandedness may deserve further study. An anomalous endocrine environment in pregnancy might modify the later hormonal characteristics of the individual, and these might affect immune competence. Another possibility derives from the known effect of sex hormones on the development of certain hypothalamic nuclei, in view of the fact that several recent studies suggest that the hypothalamus may play a role in immune responses.

A genetic question that has been raised repeatedly is whether those with anomalous dominance might have a different complement of HLA haplotypes from those with standard dominance. The fact that some disorders are so strongly associated with certain haplotypes (for instance, B27 with rheumatoid spondylitis) has led to the frequent presumption that all immune disorders will have such associations. It is, of course, possible that certain haplotypes will be found in elevated frequency in those with anomalous dominance. Even if this were the case, this should not be regarded as incompatible with our hypothesis. Since most of those with a particular haplotype do not develop immune disorders, the hormonal atmosphere in utero or in early postnatal life may still play a major role. Furthermore, the HLA genes must exert their effects through particular chemical products. As we will discuss later, Ivanyi (1978) has shown that certain loci in the major histocompatibility complex of chromosome 17 of the mouse affect several different aspects of testosterone production and action.

It must also be kept in mind that particular haplotype associations have not been demonstrated for several immune disorders; the data for lupus erythematosus, for instance, are not viewed as convincing by many investigators. In addition, immune disorders occasionally occur in families in which affected members share the same haplotype, which is not found in high frequency in other individuals or other families. This suggests that a given haplotype may be important only in combination with other factors.

There is still another type of association of HLA haplotypes with immune disorders that does not necessarily entail an elevated frequency of any particular haplotype. Since the fetus receives one chromosome 6 (which carries the HLA groups) from the mother, it will share at least half its haplotypes with her. If the parents share haplotypes, then the proportion of haplotypes shared by mother and fetus will, on the average, be even higher. It has been shown both in experimental animals (Beer and Billingham 1976) and in humans

(Faulk 1981; Taylor and Faulk 1981) that the greater the degree of haplotype sharing between parents the higher the rate of infertility and fetal loss. In addition, Faulk (1981) has shown that certain disorders of the offspring are associated with an elevated rate of parental haplotype sharing. Whether shared haplotypes are most frequent in parents of children with anomalous dominance has not yet been determined.

9.3 Learning Disabilities and Immune Disorders

The data concerning the association of immune disorders with left-handedness make it possible to reevaluate certain findings in the literature on developmental learning disorders. In addition to the reports mentioned earlier of increased frequency of allergies among stutterers, celiac disease among autistic children and autoimmune thyroid disorders in their parents, and migraine among childhood dyslexics, a high frequency of food allergies (Tryphonas and Trites 1979) and atopic disorders (Geschwind and Behan 1984) have been reported among hyperactive children.

These data have been interpreted in various ways. It is sometimes assumed that the frequency of these diseases is the result of stress on children with learning disorders. However, this could not explain all the findings, such as the increased frequency of thyroid autoimmunity among unaffected parents of autistic children. Nor could it explain the apparent, although not yet adequately documented, tendency of certain disorders to be associated with each other, for instance, allergy with stuttering and bowel disorder with autism. Another explanation attributes the learning disorder to the immune disorder. On this view, for example, "celiac autism" reflects the assumption that autism might in some cases be a manifestation of celiac disease. Similarly, it has been proposed that hyperactivity may be a manifestation of food allergy.

These phenomena can be readily explained. Stuttering, autism, and childhood dyslexia are male-predominant conditions with elevated rates of nonrighthandedness, in which one would expect high rates of immune disorders both in patients and in relatives. A concordant observation is that autistic children have a high frequency of relatives with Down syndrome (Coleman 1976), a condition with an elevated rate of thyroid autoimmunity. Against the common assumption that autoimmunity in Down patients is a secondary result of chromosomal abnormality is the finding that the parents, who have no chromosomal abnormality, also have an elevated rate of thyroid autoimmunity (Fialkow 1964, 1970). Furthermore, in Down syndrome the posterior portion of the superior temporal gyrus is commonly found to be thin (Greenfield et al. 1958); in other words, there is a disturbance of the same region in which disorders of neuronal migration or assembly have been found in childhood dyslexics (Galaburda and Kemper 1979; Galaburda 1983). Fialkow (1964, 1970) presents evidence that the chromosomal abnormality in Down syndrome is not the cause of the autoimmunity but possibly secondary to it.

9.4 Familial Patterns

In this section we will suggest some tentative general principles concerning familial patterns and possible directions for research. On inspection of family trees we have found that lefthandedness, learning disorder, immune disorder, and certain talents may all be present in single individuals, or they may be distributed among different family members. Thus, one nonrighthanded individual with a learning disorder and high artistic talents suffered from severe immune disorder. Throughout his family were to be found migraine, artistic talents, nonrighthandedness, and different learning and immune disorders, sometimes in the same individual and sometimes not. Another example is a strongly lefthanded childhood dyslexic with a righthanded brother and a grandmother each with a different immune disorder. In childhood autism this is a familiar pattern, since the patients themselves are often lefthanded and have a high rate of some type of malabsorption syndrome, whereas the unaffected parents and siblings have rates of autoimmune hypothyroidism (Coleman 1976) and (although this is controversial) a high rate of superior talents. Although genetic mechanisms are obviously at play, there is also a considerable degree of freedom from genetics. Although family members may share common genetic susceptibilities, many other factors, both genetic and nongenetic, modify the expression in any one individual. The family patterns illustrate a point made earlier, that influences that lead to high talents in one individual may in excess lead to serious disabilities in others. The disabilities tend to persist, since the overall Darwinian fitness of the group carrying the appropriate predisposition is high because of the production of individuals of exceptional talent.

In this chapter we have dealt with a few of the associations of anomalous dominance. In later chapters we will discuss other features that we believe to be more common in the anomalous dominance population, including certain patterns of hair color, skeletal and other anomalies, certain alterations in the vestibular system, some psychiatric conditions, and other types of special autoimmune effects. We will discuss the possible role of asymmetrical migration from the neural crest in the genesis of some of these anomalies.

10   Anomalous Dominance
        and Special Talents

According to our hypothesis, slowed growth within certain zones of the left hemisphere is likely to result in enlargement of other cortical regions, in particular the homologous contralateral area but also adjacent unaffected regions. The influences that favor anomalous dominance may thus favor talents associated with superior development of certain regions either in the right hemisphere or in adjacent parts of the left hemisphere. Even with excessive retardation of growth and the resultant migration abnormalities and learning disorders, high talents may exist as a result of compensatory enlargement of other cortical regions.

Several types of data are compatible with these conclusions. Some studies have claimed that the average level of spatial talents is higher in males (Buffery and Gray 1972). Hier and Crowley (1982) found that congenitally hypogonadal males, who lack testosterone, typically had superior verbal scores and low scores on tests of spatial function, unlike normal males. In Turner syndrome, in which there is a marked lack of all hormones, inferior spatial talents are commonly found, though verbal talents are sometimes superior. Taylor (1976, 1981) found that male temporal lobe epileptics with alien tissue (areas of disturbed neural development) in the *left* hemisphere typically had low verbal scores and high spatial scores; males with alien tissue on the right displayed the reverse pattern. This study provides evidence that in males prenatal influences may be more important than post-natal, since males with mesial temporal sclerosis, a postnatally acquired lesion, tended to show patterns similar to those of alien tissue patients, although the effects were less striking. The results in females support the view that postnatal influences may be somewhat more important in them than in males. Females with mesial temporal sclerosis tend to show greater discrepancies in verbal and performance scores, depending on the side of the lesion, than do those with alien tissue.

Other data support a role for hormonal influences on laterality and associated skills. Females with late menarche tend to have higher spatial scores than those with early menarche (Waber 1981).

Several studies have shown an elevated rate of nonrighthandedness in certain occupations, several of which require an increased use of spatial talents (Peterson and Lansky 1980): among professional athletes (McLean and Ciurczak 1982), artists (Peterson 1979), architects (Peterson and Lansky 1974), and engineers (Peterson and Lansky 1974), although there are some disagreements (Oldfield 1969). A group of particular interest includes mathematicians and the mathematically gifted, among whom there is also an increased rate of lefthandedness (Annett and Kilshaw 1982; Kolata 1983). Nonrighthanded individuals are superior on several tests of musical ability (Deutsch 1978). Some other papers show an elevated rate of nonrighthandedness in musicians (Peterson 1979; Byrne 1974; Quinan 1922), although there is disagreement (Oldfield 1969). One potential objection can be raised against these studies. In order to prove that nonrighthanded individuals are found in specially high frequency in occupations requiring high spatial talents, it would be necessary to document a low proportion of such individuals in other occupations. It might otherwise be postulated that nonrighthanded individuals are overrepresented in all populations with high talent, which is a possible interpretation of the existing data. It could be the case that although growth of the left hemisphere is slowed to a greater extent in lefthanders than in righthanders, it may attain a greater final size in lefthanders. This could occur when the growth period is prolonged— for instance, when pregnancy is longer than average or when puberty is late, which would allow for further development in childhood. This situation would be analogous to that of the greater final average height of males despite their slower rate of bone growth. Lefthanders might thus be found in increased numbers in all occupations demanding high talent, including those in which verbal talents are necessary. On the other hand, when full development was not achieved because of excessive retardation of growth, early termination of pregnancy, or early puberty, lefthanders might display developmental derangements such as learning disorders, and in more extreme cases a distinctly inferior overall level of functioning. Those with anomalous dominance could thus be present in excess both at the higher and at the lower ends of the scale of accomplishment. The very high frequency of lefthandedness in cases of mental retardation (Hicks and Barton 1975) would be consistent with this hypothesis. The data necessary for settling these questions are not yet available, however.

A related issue is that of superior talents in association with childhood learning disorders. There are, of course, many individual examples of such cases. Although some autistic children have widespread impairments, others exhibit dramatically isolated islands of superior behavior, as did an autistic girl who at the age of four displayed remarkable artistic talents. Many idiot savants illustrate this phenomenon (Sano 1918). High right hemisphere talents are common in dyslexics and in their families (Gordon 1980, 1983).

Much research is needed before it will be possible to assert confidently the existence of a "pathology of superiority," that is, compensatory growth leading to superior development of some portions of the brain as a result of poorer development of others. Goldman-Rakic and Rakic (1984) showed that if a cortical area is removed from one hemisphere of a fetal monkey, the result is hypertrophy both of the corresponding area on the opposite side and of areas in the lesioned hemisphere adjacent to the ablated region (see figure 10.1). It seems likely that at the time of cell death there is competition not only between homologous contralateral regions but also between regions in the same hemisphere.

The situation in which there is delayed development of a cortical region in one hemisphere is not necessarily equivalent in all cases to the ablation of a region. If the delaying influence acts only during the development of a particular cortical area, then one might expect hypertrophy of adjacent regions; in other words, this situation would resemble the one in which a surgical lesion is placed in that area. On the other hand, if the retarding influence is present over a longer period, it may affect other areas in the same hemisphere and thus might diminish or prevent the hypertrophy of adjacent areas, although contralateral hypertrophy should still take place and indeed might even be enhanced.

The possibility of hypertrophy of areas adjacent to a zone of retarded growth may help to explain another of the apparently paradoxical findings in childhood dyslexia. In the adult, acquired Gerstmann syndrome (acalculia, agraphia, right-left difficulty, and disordered finger identification) is almost always the result of a lesion in the left temporoparietoöccipital (TPO) junction region (Strub and

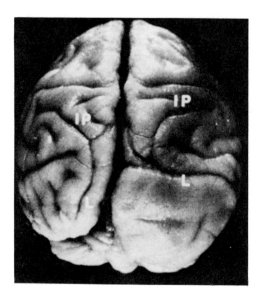

Figure 10.1
Experimental production of cortical asymmetry in the monkey (Goldman-Rakic and Rakic 1984). The left occipital lobe was resected on embryonic day 83. There is marked reorganization of fissures and sulci, and the left inferior parietal lobule is nearly twice as large as its mate on the right. *IP*, intraparietal sulcus; *L*, lunate sulcus. Reprinted by permission of the authors and Harvard University Press.

Geschwind 1974). It may exist in isolation but is usually associated with signs of involvement of adjacent regions, for instance, alexia with agraphia and constructional disorders. Some years ago Hermann (1959) reported cases of developmental dyslexia with Gerstmann signs. The dyslexic patient studied by Galaburda and Kemper (1979) had elements of Gerstmann syndrome. However, cases of developmental Gerstmann syndrome without dyslexia have also been reported by Kinsbourne and Warrington (1963) and by Benson and Geschwind (1970), the latter describing a 14-year-old boy with severe Gerstmann syndrome who had learned to read precociously and whose current reading abilities were distinctly superior for his age and grade level.

The apparent paradox may have a simple solution. As we have pointed out, the brains of several childhood dyslexics have shown disordered cytoarchitectonic organization at the TPO junction in a region known from studies of adults suffering from alexia with agraphia to be of major importance for reading (Déjerine 1891; Benson and Geschwind 1969). If the developmental disturbance should extend further into the TPO region, one might expect to find con- genital Gerstmann syndrome. If, on the other hand, the disturbed cortical architecture was clearly restricted to the region involved in reading (perhaps because adverse influences were present only over a limited period), then the immediately adjacent region might hyper- trophy. Instead of Gerstmann syndrome the affected individual might display superiority of the functions subserved by this region.

This hypothesis immediately suggests certain experiments. Among dyslexics one might find a higher proportion with superior "Gerst- mann talents" than among controls, as well as a higher proportion with poor abilities of this type than among controls. A simple assess- ment of the mean scores on tests of these abilities might obscure the elevated frequency of dyslexics at both extremes. In particular, this type of study might help in accounting both for the claim that a disproportionately high number of dyslexics exhibit high mathemat- ical ability and for the claim that a disproportionately high number of dyslexics exhibit poor mathematical ability. Both statements could be correct.

Conversely, if the major impact of deficient development fell on the "Gerstmann region," the area particularly important for reading be- ing spared, one might expect a syndrome like that of the boy de- scribed earlier who displayed Gerstmann syndrome with superior reading abilities. A related and perhaps identical problem is that of the child with very poor spelling and writing abilities in the face of high reading scores. It is often assumed that all such individuals were dyslexic at one time, but there are examples in which this appears not to be the case. The type of mechanism discussed here might account for this situation. If this interpretation is correct, then the poor spell- ers and writers should usually perform poorly on right-left, calcula- tion, and finger identification tests. (Clearly, this discussion may be relevant to the difficult problem of subtypes of dyslexia. Since this problem lies outside the scope of our book, however, we will not pursue it here.)

Sano (1918) described in detail the brain of the "genius of Earlswood" (an English institution for the mentally retarded), who, in the face of marked retardation in the development of speech and reading, had highly developed artistic abilities, especially in sculp- ture. In comparison to control cerebra, this brain had very small fron- tal lobes and small temporal lobes, but the occipital regions were massively developed. The findings are compatible with intrauterine reorganization. Interestingly, the patient's brother had a similar pattern of talents and deficits.

Though the idiot savant behavior pattern is found in some autistic children, the majority do not exhibit such spectacular islands of performance. In fact, the existence of even a small number of such cases would be unexpected in view of the great obstacles faced by these patients. Cases of this type could easily be overlooked if one simply averaged the scores of many autistic individuals. The mean level of performance has little significance in relation to a population with an excess of members at both the upper and the lower ends of the distribution.

The existence of such distributions may explain some apparently discrepant findings. Despite the finding by Peterson and Lansky (1974, 1980) that a disproportionately high number of male architects are lefthanded, several recent studies of college students found that lefthanded males scored lower on tests of spatial function than righthanded males (Berman 1971; Miller 1971). The apparent contradiction in the findings concerning spatial talents of lefthanders might be resolved if they were found in excessive numbers at both high and low levels of spatial function. We have already considered one mechanism that might account for these findings. Another type of explanation deserves brief consideration as well. Spatial performance may not be related in a simple linear fashion to the magnitude of the male-related effect in development; there may be a U-shaped relationship, with an optimal hormonal level for spatial function. On the average, the effects tend to favor the male population. On the other hand, excessive effects would also occur predominantly in males, who would therefore be found in excess number both among those with high spatial function and among those with low spatial function. The effects are less likely to reach an excessive degree in females, so that few would be in a dosage range that would lead to diminution of function. Lefthanded females might thus be found in excess in the group with high scores for spatial talent but not in the group with low scores.

It is difficult to carry out experimental studies on the problem in humans, but the existence of high spatial function in male rats, which depends on the right posterior hemisphere (Sherman et al. 1980), and the existence of anatomical asymmetries in these animals (Diamond, Dowling, and Johnson 1981; Diamond 1984; Sherman and Galaburda

1982), which can be modified by early hormonal treatments, may make controlled experimentation possible.

The possible existence of bimodal effects (that is, the findings of excessive numbers of nonrighthanded individuals at both extremes of the spectrum of certain talents) is not surprising from the perspective of biological fitness. If two populations share the same *mean* level of performance of some function, the two groups are not necessarily equally competitive. Assume that one population contains a higher percentage than the other of individuals with both very high and very low talents for this function. The population with higher numbers in the extreme ranges may compete more effectively, since success often depends primarily on the performance of those in the highest ranges. If 0.2% of the individuals in one population were talented athletes, as compared with 0.1% of the individuals in a comparable population, the first group would carry off most of the prizes. It would make no difference whether the mean level of performance of the first population was lower than that of the second or whether it also contained an excessive number of athletically untalented people. A process affecting brain growth that produced high talents in a large number, at the expense of creating an unusual number of incompetents, would be favored in the course of evolution. A mechanism of this type might not readily be detected, because of the small numbers of individuals in the tails of the distributions. An analogous situation exists in the study of the rates of chemical reactions. It was originally believed that the rates were proportional to the mean velocities of the molecules involved. It later became clear that only those molecules with velocities above a certain level (the activation energy) participate in a given reaction. It is therefore the tails of the distributions that are important. As long as the theory of reaction rates confined itself to mean velocities, no adequate theory could be constructed.

Another factor, often overlooked in the study of spatial function, may lead to erroneous conclusions. It is often assumed that spatial talent depends only on right hemisphere function, but in fact each hemisphere contributes. Left hemisphere lesions affect predominantly the placement of internal details, whereas right hemisphere lesions tend to affect external configuration. It is possible that some individuals may have high talents in one or the other function, although some are good at both. Tests of spatial function often do not distinguish these capacities, just as handedness tests may fail to distinguish pyramidal and axial motor dominance. The possibility of dissociation in spatial function is suggested by some data cited earlier; recall, for example, the dyslexic who was clumsy in trunk movements but skilled as a metalsmith. A metalsmith might need both superior small detail spatial function and high pyramidal talents, whereas an athlete might require excellent capacity for large spatial relationships and superior axial dominance. A study by Waber (1976) suggests that in early development females may have superior small detail spatial function and males may have superior capacities for large spatial relationships.

Although these patterns have unfortunately not yet been studied in adequate detail, some dyslexics appear to be superior in small detail spatial functions, whereas others are superior in the large ones such as athletic activity. If this were true, it would suggest that in some cases delayed development of the speech region leads to superior development of the adjacent posterior region in the same hemisphere, whereas in others the opposite side enlarges. Whether these differences might result from variations in timing or duration of the delaying influences, or from other factors, is not known.

Animal studies of spatial function probably tap the capacities for spatial orientation, such as those used in maze running. If left-sided dominance for small details could be shown in animals, the probability for rapid clarification of these issues would be greatly increased.

11

Sex Hormone Influences
on Brain Growth

11.1 Fetal Chromosomes and Sex Hormones

One of the major contributions of the Darwinian theory was its eluci-
dation of the importance of sexual reproduction. Although asexual
reproduction is found in many species, sexual reproduction is the
exclusive form in others, as for instance in all mammals. Since natural
selection depends on differences between animals, evolutionary
mechanisms that favor diversity have attained central importance. By
its mixing of parental genes, sexual reproduction is the most important mechanism for achieving diversity, although not the only one. It
has been known for years that sex hormones play a major role in
male-female differentiation, but until recently their effects on neural
development have received little attention. The rapid growth of
knowledge of these mechanisms has created a revolution in the brain
sciences, although they are still frequently neglected.

At fertilization the male and female zygote differ on the average in
only two chromosomes. Yet these chromosomal differences at conception are the prime movers, the ultimate origin, of all of the striking
differences in male and female development. Only the male zygote
has a Y chromosome, and it carries only one X chromosome to the
female's two.

The Y chromosome is unusual in bearing few genes; however, it
carries a protein, the H-Y antigen (Haseltine and Ohno 1981), which
is essential for development of the testes, which will later in fetal life
secrete testosterone. This hormone is, in turn, essential for the development of typically male structures in the body and brain. But H-Y
antigen does not exert all its effects only indirectly through the formation of testes and the later production of testosterone; this antigen is
expressed in other organs as well, among them the thymus gland,

an essential component of the developing immune system (Ivanyi 1978). The ovaries appear to play a more limited role in prenatal development.

The significance of the presence of one X chromosome in the male zygote and of the two in the female is sometimes underestimated because of lyonization (the random inactivation of one X chromosome in each cell of the female). In fact, inactivation does not take place in germ cells. Thus, at conception the female zygote carries twice as many X-linked genes as the male. The X chromosome plays an important role in effects of testosterone, since it contains the Tfm locus, one of the genes that controls sensitivity to this hormone (Bardin and Catterall 1981). Thus, although the female conceptus is usually exposed later in gestation to a lower level of testosterone than the male, it is probably more sensitive to maternally and placentally produced testosterone, especially in the earliest stages of embryogenesis. At the time of lyonization one might expect the embryo to lose this higher sensitivity, but inactivation is not complete and the female retains a greater dosage of some X-linked products (Naftolin 1981).

H-Y antigen is essential for the formation of testes. It is intriguing that both the right testis and the right ovary develop before the gonad on the left, and development of the ovary occurs somewhat later than that of the testis (Mittwoch 1975). The development of the testes is of cardinal importance for later development. The male fetal gonads produce testosterone in high quantities; in fact, at times the fetal level is comparable to that of adult males. The rate drops late in pregnancy and even more shortly after birth; it rises again for several months and then declines, only to rise yet again as puberty approaches. Testosterone and its metabolites are essential not only for normal development of genitalia and secondary sexual characteristics but also for the formation of the brain. Sex hormones affect the development of nervous structures involved in the control of reproduction, for instance, the cyclic release of gonadotropins, mating, and lactation. But hormones also affect body and brain systems in ways other than those related directly to reproduction. Males and females differ in almost every aspect of visible body structure, but there are also differences that transcend obvious structural features, such as gender-related variations in the immune system, in responsiveness to drugs and toxins (Selye 1971) and in metabolism (Gustaffson et al. 1978).

Before the testes begin to produce testosterone, most aspects of the hormonal environment are the same for male and female fetuses. The mother and the placenta produce great quantities of estrogens, progesterone, and gonadotropins. The fundamental pattern of the mammal is female, and specific influences must supervene in order to produce male differentiation. As development advances, the number of sex differences increases. Thus, although testosterone has a special role as a prime mover, the eventual pattern of possible influences becomes increasingly complex. The female zygote is also exposed to testosterone, little or none of which appears to come from the fetal ovaries or adrenals, but which comes instead from the maternal ovaries, adrenals, and extragonadal structures such as fat. The fetus is protected from much of this maternal testosterone, because aromatase in the placenta converts it to estradiol, but the protection is not complete.

The level of ambient testosterone is not the only factor determining testosterone effect. Testosterone-binding globulin (TeBG) lowers the level of active free testosterone. Furthermore, the sensitivity of target tissues may vary. In the syndrome of testicular feminization male fetuses produce testosterone but are insensitive to it. In addition, the rates of reaction in metabolic pathways that can inactivate testosterone probably vary considerably. Thus, although male and female zygotes differ on the average in the degree of testosterone effect to which they are subjected, there is no absolute difference between the sexes. There is evidence that testosterone in small amounts may be essential for some aspects of normal female differentiation in the rat (Dohler 1978).

Another significant hormone is progesterone, which is also present in large amounts during fetal life and is known to have masculinizing effects in the female, at least at certain periods. Sensitivity perhaps differs in the two sexes. Many of the effects of testosterone may, of course, be mediated indirectly. Biegon and McEwen (1982) have found male-female differences in serotonin systems, which might play a special role in laterality. It is worth noting that infants of mothers who have taken LSD (a serotonin derivative) in pregnancy may have missing fingers, especially on the right hand (Assemany, Neu, and Gardner 1970), which also suggests that serotonin may play a role in laterality. As we will point out later, serotonin derivatives can produce asymmetrical pharmacological effects in adults.

11.2 Hormonal Effects on Brain Structure

Since the 1960s knowledge has grown rapidly concerning the role of early sex hormone exposure in determining later sexual behavior (Naftolin 1981). This remarkable literature has shown the importance of such hormonal effects for the development of normal cycling in the female, for determining the nature of the sex object, and for other aspects of sexual and maternal behavior. It is not possible to review this vast literature in its entirety, but we will present some of the important principles. It should be noted that despite many common features, no single set of mechanisms will be universally applicable in all species (McEwen 1981). Knowledge concerning the details of the process in the human is, of course, limited. Research on sex hormone effects on neural development has dealt primarily with structures in the hypothalamus and limbic system controlling sexual behavior in the rat. Much of it has focused on the effects of sex hormones in the immediate postnatal period, when the rat is comparable to a human fetus still within the uterus in late pregnancy, but even in the rat many important developments take place before parturition. Denef (1976) has shown that the masculinization of the sexually dimorphic ventromedial nucleus of the hypothalamus begins prenatally but continues after birth. Although the human brain at birth is relatively more advanced than that of the rat, recent findings suggest that in the postnatal period, even perhaps up to puberty, important changes, including extensive cell death, are taking place in the human brain (Huttenlocher 1979).

Many locations in the nervous system contain receptors for the gonadal hormones, including estradiol and testosterone (Stumpf et al. 1976). The effects of hormones may be modulated by other influences; for instance, some actions of estradiol in certain locations such as the liver require the presence of prolactin. Furthermore, not all estrogens or androgens will necessarily exert similar effects at a particular site. Dihydrotestosterone, the metabolite that affects many of the secondary male characteristics, does not act in some species in certain locations in the nervous system in which only testosterone may be effective. The actions of testosterone itself vary from location to location within the brain. Certain neurons within the rat preoptic nucleus and amygdala contain aromatase, the enzyme that converts testosterone to estradiol. The action of testosterone within the preoptic nucleus in the rat depends on this conversion. There are other locations in which aromatase is not found, even though the target organ contains testosterone receptors; one of these is the pituitary gland.

The sex hormone receptors in the cortex are, of course, of special interest to us. Estradiol receptors are present in the cortex in the postnatal rat, but apparently not in adult life, and the same is true for enzymes involved in steroid metabolism, thus suggesting that sex hormone effects are prominent only during a certain period of development (Kolodny 1984). In particular, it should be noted that the rat cortical neurons do not contain aromatase. According to P.S. Goldman-Rakic (personal communication), however, estradiol and testosterone receptors have recently been found in association cortex of infant monkeys, along with aromatase.

The development of the preoptic nucleus, essential for cyclic release of gonadotropins, is particularly interesting, since this nucleus has a distinctly different structure in the adult male and female rat (Raisman and Field 1971). The nucleus of the male is larger and contains more neurons than that of the female. If the newborn female is exposed to a single large dose of testosterone before the 15th day of postnatal life, the nucleus assumes the typical male pattern; in a male castrated at birth it retains the female pattern. The sexual dimorphism of this nucleus thus depends on the early hormonal environment. When the female form of the nucleus is present, gonadotropins are released cyclically, regardless of whether the animal is a genetic male or female, but when the male form is present, cyclic gonadotropin release does not occur.

The literature now routinely distinguishes *masculinization* from *defeminization*. A masculinizing effect is one that leads to male-typical behavior in the female, such as mounting other females. A defeminizing effect is one that leads to loss of female-typical traits, such as cyclic release of gonadotropins. The two classes of effect can occur independently, and they depend on hormonal effects at different sites. For convenience, we will use the term *masculinization* to mean "masculinization and/or defeminization" except when the distinction is critical to the discussion.

The action of testosterone in altering the structure and function of the preoptic nucleus depends critically on the presence of aromatase, which converts it to estradiol, the intracellular action of which is responsible for the change of structure and function to the male form. One might expect the nucleus to be masculinized in both males and females, since it is exposed during intrauterine life to massive levels of estradiol. In the case of the rat the widely accepted explanation is that circulating alphafetoprotein binds estradiol and thus keeps it from crossing the blood-brain barrier and reaching the neurons of the preoptic nucleus. Testosterone, not significantly bound by alphafetoprotein, can reach the nucleus, where it is converted by aromatase to estradiol, which then alters the pattern of the cells. The binding to alphafetoprotein also explains another apparently paradoxical phenomenon. The administration of diethylstilbestrol (DES), a powerful estrogenic substance, to the newborn female rat also produces masculinization of the function and structure of this nucleus. DES binds only weakly to alphafetoprotein and can therefore reach the neurons of the preoptic nucleus, where it acts like estradiol to masculinize structure and function.

Since the binding of estradiol to alphafetoprotein is not complete, some estradiol may enter the nucleus. The administration of very large amounts of estradiol can thus also produce masculinizing effects, presumably because the binding capacity of the ambient alphafetoprotein is exceeded. Pellets of estradiol implanted directly in the nucleus have the same effects.

The multiplicity of mechanisms is illustrated by the finding of Breedlove and Arnold (1980) that the male form of a sexually dimorphic nucleus in the rat spinal cord is produced by either testosterone or dihydrotestosterone, but not estradiol.

11.3 Sex Hormone Effects on the Human Brain

The situation in the human is less clear-cut (Baum 1968). First, the sexual dimorphism of the preoptic nucleus, which is so evident in the rat, is not clear in the human. Second, the human form of alphafetoprotein does not bind estradiol significantly. Humans do, however, have a sex-hormone-binding globulin that binds testosterone more powerfully than it does estradiol. Third, the effects of early exposure to androgens in the human are not as dramatic as those seen in the rat. Early exposure to androgens in adequate dosage prevents the appearance of an estrus cycle in the female rat. Human females with congenital adrenal hypertrophy who produce excessive amounts of androgens are masculinized in infancy, yet they may have essentially normal sexual function in later life.

For these reasons some have argued that the effects of early androgens in humans are totally different from their effects in the rat. This extreme view is contradicted by others who argue that the effects in the human are in the same direction, although milder. In reviewing the literature, Karsch, Dierschke, and Knobil (1973) point out that in both nonhuman primates and humans administration of testosterone in pregnancy fails to alter normal ovarian cyclicity in female offspring, but that in these cases there is pronounced morphological and behavioral masculinization. Female mice with early exposure to androgens show permanent alterations in their responses to these substances; for example, when testosterone is administered again to them in adult life, they may show increased aggressiveness in contrast to normal adult females (Edwards 1964; Bronson and Desjardins 1968). Money and Ehrhardt (1972) have found that human females with congenital adrenal hypertrophy do show differences from other females later on, for instance, an increased tendency to participation in rough and tumble sports. Although many of these women marry and bear children, studies must still be carried out on large series to determine whether they suffer changes in menstrual function, fertility, and pregnancy.

Further evidence supports the view that changes in the human are similar to those in the rat, although of lesser degree. For reasons given above, DES in the female rat resembles testosterone in its central actions; females exposed early have abnormal estrus function in adult life and increased sensitivity to the actions of androgens. Although the majority of human females exposed to DES resemble other women on the average, certain features are more common in this population; for example, DES has been shown to have masculinizing effects on the structure of the genitalia (Bongiovanni, Di George, and Grumbach 1959). DES daughters have been reported to have an elevated rate of menstrual difficulties, infertility, and problems during pregnancy, including premature and preterm births, prolonged labor, and a higher rate of children with congenital anomalies (Herbst et al. 1980), though agreement on this is not universal. However, it should be noted that the mothers of these women also had some of these problems, which probably constituted the reason for their taking DES. It will be necessary to study a large number of DES daughters in order to ascertain whether they show an increased rate of the changes in the cortex that we have hypothesized would result from high intrauterine testosterone exposure. One might expect DES daughters to have an elevated frequency of lefthandedness, learning disabilities, high spatial talents, and the other associations hypothesized to be more frequent with elevated intrauterine male-related effects. Hines (1982) has reviewed the effects of DES. We have carried out a study on a group of 77 adults exposed to DES in utero, and our preliminary results show a markedly elevated rate of non-righthandedness in this population. Nichols and Chen (1981) have found that sex hormones administered to pregnant women lead to an elevated rate of hyperactivity in the offspring, especially in the girls.

11.4 Sex Hormone Effects on Cortex

Evidence exists to support the possibility that sex hormones might affect cortical structure. Diamond, Dowling, and Johnson (1981) have found that in the male rat at birth, and in later life, the cortex of several areas in the posterior right hemisphere is significantly thicker than in corresponding areas on the left. By contrast, females tend to have thicker areas on the left at the same periods. If the male is castrated at birth, many of the differences in favor of the right side are not observed at 90 days of age (Diamond 1984); castration of the newborn female also alters its typical pattern. In addition, ovarian hormones administered at birth alter the later pattern of cortical asymmetries. These data clearly support a role for sex hormones in postnatal development in the rat, in this case for both ovarian and testicular hormones. No studies of prenatal hormone effects on rat cortical structure are known to us.

Rosen et al. (1983) have reported that prenatal testosterone alters cerebral laterality, as measured by tail posture at birth, in Wistar rats. Female pups show a predominance of tail turning to the left, whereas males show little lateral preference. Prenatal testosterone causes a shift of the tail posture to the right in female pups but has no significant effect on males. This work, however, needs replication.

Glick (1983) has studied the turning tendencies of Sprague-Dawley rats. In litters with an excess of males there is an increase in the number of females rotating to the left, whereas in litters with an excess of females the reverse is seen. One possible explanation is that higher ambient levels of testosterone in male-predominant litters increase left-turning in females. In these studies the males are unaffected by the male-female proportions in the litter. The possible effects of testosterone on human littermates will be discussed in the section on twinning.

Data in humans support the existence of hormonal influences on development of the cortex. Taylor (1969) studied cases of temporal lobe epilepsy with unilateral mesial temporal sclerosis (MTS), a lesion believed to follow febrile convulsions. Nearly all MTS patients in this series had had a first seizure before the age of five. Among patients with a first febrile convulsion before the age of one there was a predominance of males with left-sided MTS. With increasing age there were fewer new cases, and these were more equally divided between males and females and between the right and left sides. Taylor suggested that (1) seizures tend to invade less active areas in brain, (2) the right hemisphere matures before the left, and (3) maturation is faster in females than in males. Thus, the earliest cases of MTS tended to involve the least mature hemispheres, leading to a predominance of males with left-sided lesions. With increasing maturity there were fewer cases and less selectivity between males and females and between the right and left sides.

Although data on hormonal effects on cortical developments are limited, considerable data are available on direct effects of gonadal hormones on the development of neuronal assemblies in such structures as the preoptic nucleus. In most of these experiments testosterone was administered systemically. In some, however, the same effect was produced by placing hormones directly in the hypothalamus. Of particular interest is the study of Nordeen and Yahr (1983), which disclosed lateralized effects. Estradiol implanted in females on one side produced masculinization of behavior (preference for female sex objects and aggressiveness); on the other side it led to defeminization (loss of the estrus cycle). These data amplify the earlier findings of Gerendai et al. (1978), who showed that the luteinizing hormone-releasing hormone (LHRH) content of the right hypothalamus in the rat is double that of the left.

Toran-Allerand (1978) has shown direct effects of estradiol and testosterone on the growth of neurites of preoptic nucleus neurons in tissue culture. Nottebohm (1981) has provided a dramatic example of the effects of testosterone on neuronal growth in the HVc nucleus, a structure critically involved in the control of bird song. Normally only the male sings, since testosterone is required for song production; there is a striking sexual dimorphism, this nucleus being much larger in the male. The nucleus changes in size in the course of the year, growing each spring under the influence of testosterone and regressing in the fall. There is a marked functional asymmetry in this system, with dominance of the left hemisphere. No structural asymmetry has been found in HVc, however, although a modest asymmetry is found in the nucleus of nerve XII, one of the peripheral components of the song system.

There are thus many neural systems, including lateralized cortical systems in the rat and a lateralized system for singing in the bird, that are sensitive to the effects of testosterone and other sex hormones. Much more experimental evidence will be required in order to confirm the supposition that the left-sided cortical structures underlying language are particularly sensitive to this hormone in utero. The increasing availability of animal models should make it possible to ascertain whether there are significant hormonal effects on the homologues of the posterior superior temporal cortex and the adjacent junctional region of the left parietal lobe.

It is likely that there will be important species differences. The rat data suggest that there are strain differences. It is not unlikely that there will be variations in human populations in the role played by hormones. Sex hormones administered during pregnancy increased the rate of hyperactivity in the offspring, the effects being greatest in black girls and least in white boys (Nichols and Chen 1981).

Agenesis of the corpus callosum, a frequent anomaly in the BALB mouse strain, is another illustration of possible effects of hormones on cortical systems. In his original description King (1936) pointed out the great variability in the expression of this malformation. Wahlsten (1981) has clarified this perplexing situation. If a BALB female becomes pregnant while still suckling the young of a previous litter, the new litter will, on the average, contain fewer pups, a higher proportion of whom exhibit agenesis. If the female does not become pregnant until the previous litter is weaned, the new litter will, on the average, contain more pups, a lower proportion of whom are affected. At present one can only speculate on the possible causes of this remarkable phenomenon. One likely candidate for the effect of lactation on the formation of the corpus callosum is prolactin. It might have a direct effect on migrating axons, or it may alter the effects of either estradiol or testosterone on the process. It is known that in the liver certain effects of estradiol are modulated by the presence of prolactin. Another possibility is that prolactin alters immune mechanisms, which in turn affect formation of the callosum. Prolactin receptors are found on lymphocytes, and prolactin can disinhibit certain forms of suppression of the immune response (Newson-

Davis and Vincent 1982). There are, of course, other possibilities to be considered.

Although H-Y antigen is expressed on structures other than the testes—for example, on the thymus (Ivanyi 1978)—it is unlikely that it is the major mediator of sex differences in brain effects. Females do not carry H-Y antigen, but it is clear that many of the effects observed in males are observed in females, although less often, presumably because of exposure to androgens at lower levels. In addition, as noted, females may have high sensitivity to testosterone.

11.5 Other Chemical Effects on Brain Development

Even if it is true that a male-related factor modulates intrauterine growth of certain cortical regions, it is obvious that cortical development will be susceptible to many other influences, some closely related to the hormonal effects, some more remote. Ward and Weisz (1980) showed that if a female rat is stressed during the course of pregnancy, the male offspring show demasculinization. After the stress there is a rapid rise of testosterone in male fetuses, followed by a fall to subnormal levels. It is not clear exactly how stress on the mother leads to this sequence of changes. It is interesting to note that the female offspring of such a stressed mother will also tend to have demasculinized male offspring, even though these females are not themselves stressed in pregnancy. Phenobarbital administered during pregnancy has similar effects, and the male offspring have permanently low testosterone levels. This is an example of a phenomenon already mentioned, whereby chemical effects on the fetus may produce permanent alterations in metabolism. When present in the female they can lead to a mechanism of nongenetic transmission to the following generation.

Sherman et al. (1980) have also demonstrated an environmental effect on lateralization. In studies carried out some years earlier it had been shown that brief periods of handling of newborn rats exerted permanent effects on emotionality and on other traits such as resistance to infection. In the more recent experiments it was shown that male rats who had been handled showed a greater right hemisphere lateralization in tests of emotionality and spatial performance than animals who had not been.

It should be clear that the emphasis on testosterone by those investigators who have studied sexual and reproductive traits in no way implies that it is the only possible mediator of the structural and chemical alterations that follow manipulations of its level. To be sure, a myriad of chemical reactions are altered by changes in the level of testosterone, and direct manipulation of any one of the steps involved could lead to similar effects. The same must be true ,of the effects of testosterone on cortical development.

11.6 Seasonal Effects

A corollary of our hypothesis is that hormonal effects on the brains of offspring may vary with the time of conception. The activity of the pineal gland changes seasonally with alterations in day length. As a general rule, during the dark winter months the pineal becomes active and suppresses both ovaries and testes, whereas in the summer it is inactive and sex hormone levels are higher. For this reason many animals bear young in the spring, an advantageous situation since temperature and food supplies are more suitable for survival. An example of such seasonal modulation of hormonal effects on the brain is observed in the HVc nucleus of the singing bird (Nottebohm 1981).

This description of pineal physiology is, however, somewhat oversimplified. An animal's sensitivity to light may vary through the year. Gonadal hormones may thus become activated in the spring, but as a result of loss of sensitivity to light over the summer hormone levels may diminish as fall approaches. Despite these facts, day length is a powerful influence. Thus, steers increase their weight more rapidly in the winter when artificial light is supplied to lengthen the day. This light-enhanced growth of muscle mass does not take place if the bull is castrated, suggesting that the effect of light is mediated through a rise in testosterone effect (Tucker and Ringer 1982).

Whereas seasonal breeding is the rule in many animals, humans tend to bear young in all months of the year. This does not exclude the existence of photoperiodicity in the human, but much more research is needed to prove or disprove it. If pineal effects on sex hormone levels are important, then the birth months of lefthanders, and of those with learning disorders, might not be uniform throughout the year, since fetuses conceived at different seasons might be subjected to very different hormonal environments. These effects should differ in the Northern and Southern Hemispheres and at the equator, although other factors, such as variations in the ethnic composition of populations, would also have to be considered. Data are still very sparse. Badian (1983) found that in males born in each of the six months beginning in September, the rate of nonrighthandedness was higher than that found in any of the other six months, but no clear trend was observed for female births. A possibly related and intriguing observation in the lamprey is the development of an asymmetrical pineal gland (Nieuwenhuys 1977). We will return later to the seasonal modulation of hormonal effects on brain development.

12   Sex Hormones and Immunity

We have hypothesized that the influences that affect brain lateralization also alter development of the immune system. Evidence exists that several genes in the major histocompatibility complex (MHC) of the mouse influence testosterone levels and sensitivity to it. In this chapter we will present some of this evidence in greater detail and consider further theoretical possibilities.

It is well known that immune disorders do not in general affect the two sexes equally. The prepubertal allergic disorders such as asthma, eczema, and hay fever are more likely to affect boys (Crawford and Beldham 1976), whereas after puberty the autoimmune disorders are usually, although not invariably, more common in females. Differences in immune responsiveness of males and females have been documented repeatedly. A common but perhaps too simple formulation is that females are more immunocompetent than males, as evidenced, for example, by a greater tendency to reject skin grafts. The NZB and NZB/W mouse models of autoimmunity show important sex differences, which will be mentioned later.

There is ample evidence that sex hormones have important effects on immunity, both during development and in later life. The greater involution of the thymus in males after puberty is prevented by castration. Wasi and Block (1961) studied the leukemia that occurs in rats during regrowth of the thymus after involution produced by radiation. The frequency of leukemia was diminished when radiation was followed by administration of testosterone, which inhibited thymic regrowth. Several papers document that testosterone diminishes the size of the thymus gland during development (Dougherty 1952; Frey-Wettstein and Craddock 1970). Testosterone administration leads to destruction of the bursa of Fabricius in the chick embryo (Warner, Szenberg, and Burnet 1962). Orchidectomy in the prepubertal state delays thymic involution, and the postpubertal state leads to hypertrophy (Castro 1974).

The effects of sex hormones on immunity are not confined to estrogen and testosterone. Lymphocytes have prolactin receptors (but not receptors for testosterone or estradiol), and prolactin will reverse the suppression of immune responses by suppressor T-cells (Newson-Davis and Vincent 1982; Stimson 1982). It is possible that this effect protects the nursing infant. By increasing the immune responsiveness of the mother, prolactin may heighten her resistance to infection, an effect advantageous to the nursling.

The relationship of sex hormones, especially testosterone, to immunity is an intimate one, as shown by the studies of Ivanyi (1978) on the MHC of the mouse, the group of genes that play so central a role in the control of immune responsiveness. Ivanyi found loci in the MHC that control the weight of the testis, the serum level of testosterone, the level of testosterone-binding globulin, responsiveness to testosterone, and the expression of the H-Y antigen on the thymus gland. The presence of H-Y antigen on the thymus gland suggests that this substance may play a role in male-female differences in immunity, but it cannot be the only determinant, since evidence for direct testosterone effects is plentiful. Another locus in the MHC, which controls the production of the fourth component of complement, also controls the level of sex-linked protein, a substance normally found in the male but not the female mouse. The thymic epithelium, which processes lymphocytes both in development and in later life, contains both testosterone and estradiol receptors, which have not been found on lymphocytes, according to Stimson and Crilly (1981).

There is another locus found in the human on chromosome 15, which controls production of beta-2-microglobulin (B_2M), a protein essential for immune responsiveness. Ohno (1977) has suggested that it is also necessary for the expression of the H-Y antigen, which is itself essential for the development of the male gonads. Smith et al. (1983) have reported, on the basis of large family studies, that dyslexia is linked to a locus on chromosome 15. It would not be surprising, from the point of view of our theory, if a locus that is involved in immune response and testicular development is also involved in the predisposition to dyslexia.

There are still other relationships between the sex hormones and immunity. Alphafetoprotein is an estradiol-binding protein in the rat and therefore plays a major role in the processes that lead to sexual dimorphism of the preoptic nucleus and other structures. It also possesses distinct immunosuppressant actions (Murgita and Tomasi 1975). Unfortunately, it is not clear that one can extrapolate readily from the rat to the human. Although alphafetoprotein is apparently not thought to be a sex-hormone-binding globulin in humans, there are some intriguing parallels. Alphafetoprotein is found in elevated quantities in the amniotic fluid of mothers bearing children with neural tube defects and other major anomalies of the central nervous system. Patients with Louis-Bar syndrome (ataxia-telangiectasia), who exhibit maldevelopment of the nervous system, immune disorders, and in some cases gonadal dysgenesis (Sedgwick and Boder 1972), also have a high level of alphafetoprotein.

Prolactin is another reproductive hormone with immune effects that may perhaps affect neural development. We have noted that the female BALB mouse is more likely to produce offspring suffering from agensis of the corpus callosum if her litter is conceived while she is lactating (Wahlsten 1981).

H-Y antigen is expressed on sperm and on the thymus gland (Ivanyi 1978). There are common antigens to germ cells and to brain (Golub 1982), suggesting a close developmental relationship between the two that may have important clinical reflections. Schoene et al. (1977) reported the postmortem findings of a patient who had died after a prolonged neurological illness coming on after an episode of orchitis. In addition to typical severe lesions of multiple sclerosis, the postmortem disclosed severe hypertrophic peripheral neuropathy. Another patient who had had a vasectomy developed a similar clinical syndrome. We have recently seen a third patient whose first attack of multiple sclerosis coincided with a genitourinary infection. Dr. Andrew Herzog is now preparing a report on a group of patients seen by him and by us who developed a first temporal lobe seizure following an orchitis, an epidydimitis, or other genital infection. P. Paterson (personal communication) found in experiments with S. M. Harwin that 10% of rats immunized with homogenized testis or ovary develop the histological changes of experimental allergic encephalomyelitis. The Obese (OS) chicken is a strain that develops a rapidly progressive immune thyroiditis after birth, which can be controlled by administration of testosterone (Talal 1977b). It is, of course, likely that the immune system has a special role in the development of the nervous system. A remarkable feature of the immune system is its extensive polymorphism, so that lymphocytes are produced that can recognize enormous numbers of different antigens. Ohno (1977) has suggested that this system is ideally suited to provide markers or "anchoring sites" that enable developing structures to be built in precisely the correct form. In no organ system can this type of detailed anchorage mechanism be so important as in the developing nervous system, in which many millions of nerve fibers traverse great distances and establish connections with particular groups of target cells. Marking by means of histocompatibility antigens might provide exactly such a system. Sperry (1950) showed that if a frog's eye was rotated, the nerve fibers grew back to the locations to which they would normally be connected, a finding that suggested the existence of a system of specific recognition properties. Certain viruses appear to attack neurons within connected systems, raising the possibility that the affected axons have shared anchoring sites for the virus. The poliomyelitis virus will attack the Betz cells of the primary motor cortex as well as anterior horn cells (that is, connected components of the pyramidal system), but it almost always spares the neurons controlling the extraocular muscles, the movements of which have no representation within the pyramidal system. The herpes simplex virus does not affect the nervous system randomly but tends to concentrate its attack on connected sets of neurons within the limbic system. Levitt (1984) reports that certain monoclonal antibodies bind preferentially to the different components of the limbic system.

If the immune system provides anchoring sites for the processes of axons, then sex hormones, which affect the immune system, could lead to alterations in the formation of the nervous system. If the immune system provides markers for neural development, then immune suppression at a particular period might lead to disordered neural development. These possibilities are amenable to direct experimental study.

The later occurrence of immune disorders in patients subjected to parallel influences on the thymus and nervous systems might result from diminished production of lymphocytes involved in self-recognition of certain organ systems. This suggests that the organ systems most affected would generally be those that were undergoing active development at the time of the disturbing influences on the immune system. The fact that in our studies (Geschwind and Behan 1982, 1984) the most common immune disorder found in strongly left-handed individuals involved the bowel and thyroid may given important clues to the timing of the causative events. This possibility might help to explain data mentioned earlier suggesting that particular forms of learning disability have strong associations with certain types of immune disorder.

The hypothesis that suppression of the thymus at a given period will increase the possibility of later immune attack on organs currently undergoing active development may help to explain another curious phenomenon. Certain MHC alleles in the Buffalo (BUF) rat have been found to be strongly associated with the development of autoimmune thyroiditis (Talal 1977). This raised the possibility that animals with the appropriate haplotype were more likely to produce antithyroglobulin antibodies. Yet when such antibodies were given to rats of another strain bearing the same haplotypes, they were much more resistant than BUF animals. This suggested the presence of a tissue factor, in other words, it suggested that the thyroid gland of the BUF animal was more susceptible to immune attack. Later studies have shown that the thyroids of BUF animals do indeed differ in several respects from those of nonsusceptible strains. It has also been pointed out that nonimmune thyroid disorders (such as nodular goiter) as well as immune disorders are found in elevated frequency in the families of patients with immune thyroid disease. This also suggests the presence of a tissue factor.

These findings are possible examples of the mechanism proposed above. An anomalous hormonal atmosphere at a particular period in gestation will affect both structures being formed and the processing of lymphocytes that would normally recognize those structures. This implies that malformed structures will often be susceptible to later immune attack. The malformed structure may thus be, in classical terms, a *locus minoris resistentiae* (a site of lowered resistance). The same mechanism may affect the simultaneously developing brain structures, a point to which we will return later.

The sex ratios for immune disorders may appear to present a problem, since the hypothesis implies that males should be at greater risk for immune disease. Indeed, before puberty the common immune disorders are the male-predominant allergies; after puberty the autoimmune disorders are generally, although not universally, female predominant. There is evidence, however, that testosterone in adult life acts to suppress autoimmunity, presumably by its effect on the thymus. The implication is therefore that the male is indeed *more susceptible* to autoimmune disorders but is protected by his own production of testosterone after puberty. High testosterone effect in utero increases susceptiblity to immune disease, but after puberty it diminishes its expression. If this hypothesis is correct, then males subjected to high testosterone effect in utero, but who are hypogonadal after puberty, should have very high rates of autoimmune disease. Males affected by Klinefelter syndrome appear to fit this picture, since they may have high testosterone levels even at birth but later become hypogonadal. It has been suggested that they have a high rate of autoimmune disorders.

Data on a New Zealand Black Mouse hybrid (the NZB/W) are consistent with this hypothesis. The animals develop spontaneous autoimmunity, which occurs earlier and with greater severity in the female. Castration of the female at birth has no effect, but castration of the male leads to acceleration of the immune disorder. Conversely, testosterone retards the disease in females. In another recently developed mouse model of autoimmunity males are more susceptible, but detailed hormonal studies have not yet been carried out (Theofilopoulos et al. 1983).

This hypothesis is in keeping with other findings concerning several autoimmune diseases. Myasthenia gravis is more common in young females and old men, that is, in those groups in whom androgen effects are the lowest. Lupus erythematosus has a strong female preponderance, but with increasing age the percentage of new male cases increases. Furthermore, before puberty the proportion of male cases is higher than it is after puberty. In hereditary angioneurotic edema (an immune, but not an autoimmune, disorder) one of the most effective treatments is danazol, a modified testosterone with definite, although diminished, masculinizing effects.

Many questions remain concerning the relationships between sex hormones and immunity. Not all immune disorders are female predominant; for example, Marie-Strumpell disease (rheumatoid spondylitis) is perhaps ten times as common in males as in females. It has been suggested that the female prevalence is higher than the figure just quoted because many women develop the disorder in mild form, but even if this is the case its greater severity in males must be accounted for. Furthermore, late onset female-predominant immune disorders, such as temporal arteritis, do exist. These discrepancies should not be surprising. "Immune disorder" is not a monolithic category but instead encompasses many conditions with different mechanisms. It is not unlikely that when more information is available, it will be found that certain classes of immune disorders are most frequent in lefthanders, others are most frequent in righthanders, and still others affect both types of individuals equally. In addition, sex hormones may play a large role in certain types and not in others.

Differences in the frequency of the allergic and immune diseases may well be paralleled by differences in susceptibility to infection. Females are less likely to die of infection than are males, and this must be attributable in good part to differences in the immune system. This would presumably have made excellent biological sense in earlier human communities in which the life-styles of males and females were so different. Females were more likely to be in close contact with children and other members of the community than males, who were more often away from home in open spaces. The female's resistance to infection would protect her, the children, and other members of the community. Resistance to infection may have disadvantages, since the prostrating effects of many illnesses are primarily the result of the immune response. This might have been less of a problem for females surrounded by other family members than for the more isolated males away from home. Lessened male immune response would imply less temporary incapacity, although at the price of increased risk of death from infection itself.

The possibility that decreased risk of infection is the result of a more active immune system is in keeping with recent suggestions that children susceptible to allergic disorders are more resistant to parasitic infection (Marsh, Meyers, and Bias 1981). It has been pointed out (Nussenzweig 1982) that parasitic infection tends to cause immune suppression. It would be interesting to know if this occurs less often in children susceptible to allergic disorders. This raises the question of whether males with anomalous dominance are more resistant to many infections than those with standard dominance patterns.

It is likely that some organisms will have developed special strategies for attacking individuals resistant to most infections. Even under the special conditions of pregnancy females are resistant to many infections, but they may be at elevated risk for other disorders. In the great epidemics of poliomyelitis that preceded the introduction of successful vaccination, many observers were struck by the great susceptibility of pregnant women, and the same observation was made during the worldwide spread of epidemic encephalitis in the 1920s.

Similarly, the anomalous dominance population may be resistant to most infections but more highly susceptible to others. We have been struck by an apparently high frequency of lefthandedness among former victims of poliomyelitis.

The interrelationship between laterality and the immune system is highlighted by recent findings that brain lesions in each hemiphere may have different effects on immunity. In particular, Renoux et al. (1983a,b) found that left cortical lesions in the rat reduced the number of natural killer cells, whereas right-sided lesions had no such effect.

13   Genetics and Chromosomes

13.1 Genetics of Laterality

Cerebral dominance was described long before awareness of Mendel's discoveries became widespread, but once these had entered the general scientific consciousness, investigators began to study the possible genetics of handedness. Much of the early success of the Mendelian doctrine of segregation of characters, and of the later discovery of genes, was the result of studying fairly simple systems to which the principles could be readily applied. It has become increasingly clear, however, that many phenomena can be explained only by complex mechanisms. The simplest forms of dominant or recessive transmission are easily handled, but it is more difficult to deal with polygenic inheritance. Attempts to analyze handedness on the basis of simple classical dominant or recessive inheritance were not successful. Perhaps the most successful theory of the genetics of laterality is that of Annett (1978b), which attains high agreement with observed distributions. Although our own views on the detailed genetic mechanisms involved in laterality differ from those of Annett, we must again express our debt to her contributions, without which we would have been unable to develop our own formulations. Among these important contributions is the concept of random dominance, discussed earlier. Annett postulates the existence of a gene that favors left hemisphere dominance, in the absence of which dominance for language or handedness is determined by random effects. Many pieces of evidence support this concept. Mice tend to use one forepaw consistently in a task that must be carried out unimanually, but the distribution of dextral and sinistral mice is approximately equal. Collins (1969) mated only mice who used the same paw, but after several generations of such selective breeding the offspring still showed an even distribution of dextrality or sinistrality. Clearly, these animals demonstrate random dominance for paw preference.

A similar situation prevails in hereditary situs inversus in mice (Layton 1976). Even when homozygous animals are mated, only half the offspring show reversed situs, even though the offspring with normal situs are as likely as the affected offspring to transmit the condition to their own offspring. In this case there is transmission, not of reversed situs, but rather of random situs.

Our ideas and Annett's differ chiefly in their fundamental assumptions. Annett postulates the absence of a gene for right cerebral dominance and instead the existence of one that favors a "right shift"— that is, a gene that increases the probability of left cerebral dominance for either language or handedness. Homozygotes will have an even greater probability of left cerebral dominance than heterozygotes, whereas individuals who lack the gene will have essentially random dominance. The theory specifically makes allowances for nongenetic effects, so that even among homozygotes there is an increased probability but not a certainty of left dominance. Annett's formulation successfully predicts the distribution of handedness under many conditions, although it does not deal explicitly with such phenomena as the greater degree of lefthandness in males, and in twins and their first-degree relatives.

Our own formulation in some respects resembles that of Corballis and Morgan (1978), who postulate the existence of a "left shift" (influences that tend to favor right cerebral dominance), though it also differs from theirs in several ways. We begin with the assumption that cerebral dominance is determined primarily by anatomical asymmetry, so that language lateralization will depend to a great extent on the size of the planum temporale, which is larger on the left in about 65% of brains (Geschwind and Levitsky 1968). Although the left side can be even ten times larger than the right, it is unusual for the right side to be massive compared to the left. The size distribution is markedly skewed to the left; as noted earlier, this appears to be the case even in utero (Wada, Clarke, and Hamm 1975), although the right side develops more rapidly (Fontes 1944). We presume that the basic pattern of most brains includes a larger left side. Certain influences in the course of pregnancy tend to slow development on the left; the greater these influences are, the more likely it is that the brain will be shifted toward symmetry, and in a few cases even to modest asymmetry favoring the right side. Our hypothesis is essentially the mirror image of Annett's; that is, we presume a strongly left-hemispheric basic dominance pattern, along with a set of influences producing a shift to increasing symmetry and thus favoring random dominance.

We have already described several genetic factors that might play a role in this process by controlling the levels of hormones, especially testosterone, as well as sensitivity to it. These include the Y chromosome, several major histocompatibility locus genes, and genes on the X chromosome and chromosome 15. There are probably other types of genetic influence; for example, the baseline level of left-sided asymmetry probably varies in the population.

Our hypothesis helps to explain certain aspects of the distribution of handedness that some other proposals do not account for, such as the greater frequency of lefthandedness in males. In section 13.7 we will discuss the elevated rates of lefthandedness in twins and their first-degree relatives, another feature that poses a problem for many theories.

Other features of the familial distributions present problems for any genetic theory, for example, a trend for lefthanded mothers more than lefthanded fathers to have lefthanded children. We will argue that the number of nongenetic factors involved in the determination of laterality is so large that no purely genetic theory will be able to deal with them. These factors will not affect all fetuses at random but may preferentially affect a particular group, such as males, females, or twins. Further discussion of the existing genetic theories may be found in Porac and Coren (1981) and Bryden (1982).

The difficulties inherent in this field are well demonstrated by two sets of breeding experiments. Larrabee (1906) described the asymmetry of the completely decussated optic nerves in the trout and cod; the nerve from the right eye crosses dorsal to the one from the left in 60% of cases. His attempts to alter this ratio by selective breeding failed. In an ingenious experiment he produced two-headed monsters, the two heads of which had, of course, identical genetic endowments. The distribution of right or left dorsal crossings in the two heads was identical to that found in two individuals chosen at random from the general population.

The flounder has both eyes on one side of its head. In some individuals the eyes are on the right; in others they are on the left. The distribution on the two sides varies in the different species that occupy particular geographical niches. Cross-breeding experiments between species have been carried out, with findings that do not fit readily into any standard nuclear genetic model (Policansky 1982). It is possible that variations in the distribution of asymmetry may be determined to a great extent by differing environmental conditions, such as water temperature or food supply. This possibility gains credence from the fact that the sex ratio of the offspring of certain species shifts sharply from female predominant to male predominant depending on temperature or food supply (Clutton-Brock 1982; Harvey and Slatkin 1982). In several species the sex ratio can vary considerably depending on the hormonal conditions of pregnancy. James (1980a,b) has suggested that this may be true even in humans. It is thus also conceivable that there is a genetic bias toward one form of laterality, which is modified by environmental conditions that alter hormonal milieu or the time of fertilization.

Another problem for any genetic theory of laterality is the existence of genes that may determine the presence of asymmetry but not its direction. Dahlberg (1944–47) pointed out several examples in both animals and humans. Certain unilateral anomalies such as polydactyly (more than five digits on a hand or foot) or heterochromia iridis (different colors of the two irises) may be found in different members of a kinship, sometimes on one side, sometimes on the other. This is in contrast to other unilateral anomalies, which may be consistently on one side. Dahlberg suggested the existence of genes determining asymmetry but not direction. Collins (1969) has suggested that one can breed mice for a strong tendency to use one paw, but not for which paw will be used.

13.2 Cytoplasmic and Maternal Inheritance

Why do human brains exhibit a basic pattern favoring left hemisphere dominance in the great majority of instances? In our view the most reasonable hypothesis has been advanced by Corballis and Morgan (1978), namely, that a fundamental asymmetry exists, probably in the ovum itself. This fundamental asymmetry may well be determined by maternal cytoplasmic factors, which deserve a brief discussion.

Most accounts of inheritance refer to nuclear genes, that is, genes located on chromosomes. Another group of genes, overwhelmingly maternally derived, is found in the cytoplasm. The ovum contributes many cytoplasmic genes to the zygote; the sperm contributes few, if any (Birky 1983). These cytoplasmic genes are well known in plant genetics but have received less attention in studies of animal hered-

ity. Special emphasis has been placed on cytoplasmic genes associated with mitochrondria, which has led to underscoring their role in
regulating energy metabolism within the fertilized egg before the
conceptus develops its own metabolic systems controlled by its own
nuclear genes. Recent studies show that at least in some species maternal cytoplasmic genes are also involved in production of structural
proteins such as actin (Davidson, Hough-Evans, and Britten 1982).
Furthermore, these genes may be active during development for a
much longer period than was previously thought. It is increasingly
clear that these genes are important in higher animals.

Cytoplasmic genes are often modulated by nuclear genes. In
Drosophila the inheritance of the anomaly designated as *tumor head* is
jointly controlled by cytoplasmic and nuclear genes (Jenkins 1979). A
striking example of another type of cytoplasmic role in heredity is
afforded by the snail *Limnea peregra*, the spiral patterns of whose
shells were studied by Boycott and Diver (1923–24). In the initial
studies the dextral or sinistral spiral patterns of offspring appeared to
have little relationship to those of the parents. It eventually became
clear that this was an example of *delayed inheritance*. There are nuclear
genes for dextral coiling *(d)*, which are dominant, and for sinistral
coiling *(s)*, which are recessive. The coiling of the offspring is determined *only by the mother's genotype*. Thus, if the mother carries *ds*
genes, the offspring all coil dextrally regardless of the genes contributed to the zygote by the sperm. If the father also carries *ds* genes,
this does not affect the coiling of the offspring, some of which will be
dd, others *ds*, and still others *ss*. An *ss* female offspring of this union of
two *ds* parents will herself coil dextrally, but all her offspring will coil
sinistrally. The coiling pattern of the offspring is thus determined by
nuclear genes contributed by the ovum, which control the pattern of
spiral cleavage. These nuclear genes thus act on the cytoplasm of the
zygote, possibly by affecting the expression of cytoplasmic genes.
Freeman and Lundelius (1982) have shown that the dextral gene carries a product that will cause dextral coiling if injected into the maternal cytoplasm, but the sinistral gene has no effect. Whether such
delayed effects on asymmetry are seen in higher animals and in particular in humans has not, to our knowledge, been studied.

Another way to describe these data is by pointing out that coiling of
any individual can be predicted from the genetic endowment of the
maternal grandparents. The potential application to the human is obvious. It will be important to ascertain whether this type of delayed

inheritance plays a role in humans. Another point to stress is that in the situation just discussed the mother's contribution to the offspring's laterality is more important than the father's. Several studies in humans have shown a closer relationship in laterality between offspring and mother than between offspring and father (Porac and Coren 1981).

Nance (1969) has called attention to a maternal effect in the inheritance of human neural tube defects. Mothers who had conceived an infant with a neural tube defect by one husband were more likely than control mothers to have an affected child by a second husband. By contrast, fathers of a child with a neural tube defect by one wife were no more likely than control fathers to have an affected child in a second marriage. These data suggest a maternal factor affecting neural tube development.

Although we agree with the basic postulate of Corballis and Morgan (1978) concerning a maternal cytoplasmic effect favoring the left hemisphere, we do not agree with their additional assumption that the left hemisphere grows more rapidly. The available evidence, reviewed in detail in chapter 5, clearly supports the contrary claim, that the right hemisphere develops faster than the left.

If cytoplasmic inheritance plays a role in the human, are we to assume that the ovum always carries a bias toward larger speech and handedness regions in the left hemisphere, or does some minority of ova carry a bias in the opposite direction? In the studies of Boycott et al. (1930) most female snails carried a dextral bias, and a small number carried a sinistral bias. A. C. Verkoren (personal communication) has, for example, argued that right and left biases in cytoplasmic genes may be primary determinants of laterality. If more than one bias is present in the population, are we to assume that all the ova of a particular human female carry the same bias? Although many copies of cytoplasmic genes are found in a cell, it is likely, on the basis of recent studies, that different alleles would either not be present at all or be present only in very small numbers (Birky 1983). The ova of one particular female would therefore presumably carry only a single bias. At present there is no way to deal with these questions, but the existence of asymmetry in other species should make many of them readily accessible to laboratory experimentation. We will discuss the issue of reverse bias in chapter 19. As we will point out shortly, even if such biases exist in humans, they must be modified to a considerable extent by nongenetic factors.

13.3 Paternal Effects

The father contributes half his nuclear genes to the zygote at fertilization but has no further influence on its development. Preconception environmental influences can, however, alter the paternal contribution. Some gross effects of this type are easy to understand; for example, radiation causing damage to paternal germ cells could lead to chromosomal damage and thus to effects on offspring. Some environmental effects may be less crude. A disproportionate number of parents of autistic children, both fathers and mothers, are reported to have had contact with toxic chemicals (Coleman 1976). It is possible that chemicals might preferentially affect the fertilizing capacity of sperm carrying certain specific genes. Genes on the Y chromosome could be a source of paternal influences on male offspring. It appears likely that the major effects of this chromosome are mediated indirectly via the induction of testes and the production of testosterone. There is evidence, however, that the Y chromosome may have direct genetic effects, as shown, for instance, by the work of Maxon, Ginsburg, and Trattner (1979) on the inheritance of aggressive behavior in rats.

Another possible source of paternal effects is the T/t gene complex, which is located in the major histocompatibility complex in the mouse (Andrews and Goodfellow 1982; Dunn 1964). It has been suggested that a homologue of this gene complex exists in humans, but this is still under discussion (Goodfellow and Andrews 1983). Although the mouse homozygous for the allele t does not survive, animals heterozygous for t are still found with high frequency. Although only half of the sperm of a t-bearing father carry this gene complex, t is transmitted to more than half the offspring, presumably because a sperm bearing t has a greater chance of fertilizing an ovum than one that does not. Thus, the offspring of a father heterozygous for t will inherit t in a large majority of matings. This group of genes may have a role in neural development since the nonviable tt homozygote frequently has anomalies thought by some to resemble human neural tube defects. Exposure of the father to chemicals might well alter the expression of t in sperm and thus change the proportion of offspring who carried this allele and the genes linked to it. Since t not only affects the probability of fertilization by the sperm that carries it but also inhibits recombination in the chromosome on which it is located, it could well play an important role in altering expected standard genetic effects. There is no evidence at present that t plays a role in dominance, but with the identification of dominance in rodents this possibility could be tested.

Exposure of the father to toxic chemicals might simply modify the genes transmitted to the offspring (for instance, by methylation) and thus alter the environment of the fetus. There is as yet no clear evidence for any of these speculations.

Another speculative possibility is that paternal cytoplasmic genes could be carried into the zygote. We know of little information bearing on this possibility, but most authorities on cytoplasmic inheritance tend to regard it as unlikely. Although some paternal cytoplasmic genes are probably contributed to the conceptus, their number is very small. As has been pointed out, they are likely not to play an important role in mammals (Birky 1983).

13.4 The Role of Nongenetic Factors

Annett (1978b) postulates that possession of the right-shift gene increases the probability of left hemisphere dominance; the magnitude of the effect, however, varies from individual to individual because of other random influences. One such influence might be other genes producing small modifications in the effects of a major gene.

Environmental factors can be an important source of nongenetic influences on laterality. Since the effect of a gene is to play a role in some form of chemical reaction, it is not surprising that genetic determination is not absolute. Every chemical reaction can be modified by alterations in pressure, temperature, pH, light, the presence of other substances, the availability of chemical precursors, and the rate at which products are removed. With the growing sophistication of molecular genetics, it has become increasingly clear that nongenetic effects can play a powerful role; methylation, for example, has been shown to suppress expression of many genes. We will now consider some of the random effects that might modify lateralization.

One implication of our hypothesis is that even if the genetic endowment of any particular fetus were known precisely, it would not be possible to predict the exact lateralization pattern of the brain, although it would be possible to make predictions concerning the distribution in a population basis. One of the reasons for this relative freedom from genetic determination is that if hormones do play a role in determining laterality, then the effects of testosterone or related substances on the developing brain will be modified by factors not under the control of the fetal genes. Androgens are produced not only by fetal testes and the placenta but also by the maternal ovaries, adrenals, and nonglandular tissues. The fetus can be influenced by the actions of many of the unshared maternal genes. It is reasonable to expect that if a fertilized ovum were transplanted into the uterus of an unrelated female, the final pattern of the brain would be quite different, because the brain would develop in an environment of hormones and other substances that would certainly differ in many respects.

It might therefore be reasonable to take a different approach than usual to the genetics of many conditions. One should perhaps consider, not the genes carried by the offspring alone, but rather the genes of that organism existing or active only for the nine months of pregnancy; in other words, one should consider the mother and the fetus as a unit. This unit contains three groups of different genes: one paternal set present in the fetus, one maternal set present in the mother, and another maternal set present both in the mother and in the fetus. The situation is even more complex when dizygotic twins are involved, since the maternal-fetal unit will contain another group of paternal genes.

The effects of substances produced by the mother will, however, be diminished by the capacity of the placenta to act as a barrier to some maternal hormones. The fetus is protected to a great extent from maternal testosterone, which is converted to estradiol by placental aromatase. Dihydrotestosterone, which is not aromatized and therefore crosses the placenta, is, however, usually present in the mother at much lower levels than testosterone. The protection from maternal testosterone is not complete, since offspring do show signs of masculinization when mothers are exposed to this hormone. In addition, progesterone administered to the mother may masculinize female fetuses. It is clear that the placental barrier is far from complete. Furthermore, it is likely that there are individual variations in the aromatizing capacity of the placenta.

It is conceivable that some maternal genes not shared by the offspring have greater effects on female fetuses. Thus, the testosterone to which female fetuses are exposed comes predominantly from maternal tissues, whereas males produce it themselves in high quantities. In the study of Nichols and Chen (1981) sex hormones given to mothers were associated with a higher rate of hyperactivity in female offspring than in males.

Two other random factors are stress during pregnancy, which can lead in the rat to demasculinization of male offspring, and exposure of the mother to exogenous chemicals. Phenobarbital administered in pregnancy also can cause demasculinization of male offspring, who develop permanently low testosterone production (Gupta, Yaffee, and Shapiro 1982). Exogenous sex hormones should, by our hypothesis, lead to modifications in lateralization of offspring. Nichols and Chen (1981) found that children of mothers who received sex hormones during pregnancy had an elevated rate of hyperactivity, another condition in which an elevated rate of lefthandedness is also found.

Denenberg et al. (1978) have shown a direct effect of postnatal environment on lateralization. Male rats handled in infancy exhibit more conspicuous right hemisphere lateralization of certain activities than animals who are not handled. Previous studies on early handling demonstrated a wide variety of later metabolic and hormonal alterations (Denenberg and Zarrow 1971). If metabolic effects alter dominance, then maternal diet may represent yet another nongenetic influence.

The argument thus far might be summarized by a statement made earlier: an individual could have different dominance characteristics if the fertilized ovum were transplanted into another mother's uterus. Although this hypothesis cannot be tested easily in humans, it is certainly amenable to straightforward study in experimental animals.

The time of conception is another nongenetic random variable that may well significantly influence laterality. Seasonal effects have often been considered narrowly. The fact that schizophrenics are more likely to be born in January than July, a finding documented repeatedly, has often been interpreted as a result of increased susceptibility of newborn infants to virus infection in the winter. There are many other possibilities, however. Consider, for example, changes in sex hormones with day length. The pineal gland, activated in the dark months, tends to suppress gonadal hormonal production. When it is suppressed, during periods of long days, sex hormone levels rise. We have already alluded to Badian's (1983) report of a higher rate of nonrighthandedness in males conceived from December through May (days being shortest on December 21 and increasing in length for the following six months). A pineal role in laterality has no direct experimental support, but it certainly deserves study.

Ample data confirm the importance of seasonal factors in other areas as well. Seasonal variation in congenital anomalies has been repeatedly documented. Clearly, these anomalies cannot be attributed to postnatal effects, such as susceptibility of the offspring to infection. Births of infants with neural tube defects are most common in the first three months of the year, and twin births show a similar marked seasonal variation. It is known that mothers given human chorionic gonadotropin bear a greater number of dizygotic twins. One might expect circumannual variations in sex hormone production to be paralleled by changes in the gonadotropin level, leading to more twin conceptions in the months in which maternal gonadotropin levels were the highest.

13.5 Transgenerational Effects

There is another possible but surprising source of random variation. When rats are subjected to stress during pregnancy, the offspring show altered emotional behavior. In turn, the offspring of affected female offspring show similar changes in emotional behavior despite the fact that their mothers were not exposed to any additional stress. This can readily be explained. The offspring of a mother subjected to stress in pregnancy show permanent alterations in their own behavior and are more susceptible to stress effects than normal animals. Therefore, when the females among them become pregnant, even minor stresses will affect them, and their offspring will in turn be affected—an example of what might loosely be termed a "Lamarckian" effect.

There are two mechanisms by which such persistent effects of stress could be mediated. Stress produces structural alterations in the brain of the offspring and/or permanent metabolic alterations. Thus, newborn female rats exposed to testosterone manifest a series of permanent metabolic changes. They are more sensitive in later life to androgens than normal females. They carry sex-linked protein, which is normally found only in males (Michaelson 1981), and certain liver enzymes normally found in females disappear (Gustaffson et al. 1978). There is thus an increased possibility that the female who was subjected to excessive testosterone effects in utero will herself show an increased tendency to hormonal masculinization, which will in turn affect her offspring. In the rat diethylstilbestrol (DES) has masculinizing effects on brain regions involved in reproductive behavior (MacLusky and Naftolin 1981). In the human DES also appears to have certain masculinizing effects (Bongiovanni, Di George, and Grumbach 1959); moreover, as mentioned earlier, DES daughters have been reported in some series to have a higher rate of infertility and difficulties in pregnancy, although this result is controversial (Beral and Colwell 1981). We hypothesize that these women will have a higher proportion of children with anomalous dominance, that is, a higher rate of lefthandedness and of the other associations of atypical laterality. Preliminary studies now under way appear to confirm this.

There will be certain limitations on such transgenerational masculinizing effects. Even if the mother is masculinized by endogenous or exogenous hormones, the fetus may be shielded from them to a varying degree by the placenta and by the effects of paternal genes.

13.6 Age and Parity Effects

Maternal age and parity (the number of children previously borne) both influence the outcome of pregnancy, but these two influences are often confused. In order to separate the effects, it is necessary to compare women of equal parity but different age, and women of equal age but different parity. Since the two influences might work in opposite directions, failure to separate them may cancel out any positive effects. Twinning in Nigeria increases with both age and parity (Bulmer 1970; Nylander 1978). Some congenital anomalies, such as neural tube defects, also vary with age and parity. Certain other factors thought to influence twinning or neural tube defects may be reducible to these influences.

The exact reasons for these effects are not entirely clear. It has been speculated that parity effects may depend on immune factors. An obvious example is erythroblastosis fetalis, occurring in Rh + children of Rh − mothers, which is more likely to occur in later pregnancies, since the mother is sensitized to fetal red cells in the first pregnancy and produces antibodies more rapidly in a second one. Another possibility may be that high parity selects for women who may be particularly fertile as a result of high levels of hormones. The cause of age effects is also not fully clarified, although certain chromosomal changes increase with age.

Do maternal age and parity influence the frequency of anomalous dominance in the offspring? There are many papers both supporting and opposing the hypothesis that maternal age and birth order have an influence on handedness. It is clear that maternal age and parity can have influences on the offspring, which are largely independent from genetics.

It is interesting that many clinicians believe that dyslexia is more common in adopted children, but we do not know of any definite documentation for this claim. Adopted children do include a higher proportion of the offspring of very young mothers. On the other hand, it is conceivable (though speculative) that adopted children are disproportionately often the offspring of parents with anomalous dominance. This problem deserves more careful documentation and further study.

13.7 Twins and Anomalous Dominance

Even early studies of the genetics of handedness revealed an excess of lefthanders among twins and, even more surprising, among their relatives. The recent work of Boklage (1984) has shown that the rate of lefthandedness in twins (both monozygotic and dizygotic), and in their mothers, fathers, and siblings, is double the rate in the siblings of the parents. This would appear to support the belief that twinning and lefthandedness are associated, since otherwise one would have to argue that the second-degree relatives of twins had lower rates than the general population. The elevated rate of lefthandedness in both types of twins and their first-degree relatives has no simple genetic explanation and may reflect nongenetic influences.

The distribution of lefthandedness among identical twins has typically been one of the major difficulties in the formulation of any genetic theory of handedness. One would expect that in any identical twin pair both would be righthanded or both lefthanded. Yet this is conspicuously not the case. A typical distribution might be: both righthanded, 80%; both lefthanded, 4%; one right, one left, 16%.

Annett explains this distribution by her genetic theory. A certain number of twin pairs would not carry the right-shift gene; therefore, in these pairs handedness would be random. In one-quarter of the pairs both twins would be lefthanded, in another quarter both would be righthanded, and in half there would be opposite handedness.

This is in contrast to other popular explanations, one of which is the theory that some twin pairs are mirror images. In general, this notion has not been widely accepted in recent years, in part because it is rare to find situs inversus in one member of a pair of identical twins. In experimental animals it is possible to produce twin pairs, one of which does show situs inversus, but it is still likely that this is at best a rare event among humans.

The other popular theory, which has been applied to both types of twins, is that of birth trauma. Since twins are more likely to have difficult births, the argument is advanced that it will not be rare for one twin to suffer some brain damage. As Satz (1973) has pointed out, random unilateral brain damage at birth will tend to increase the number of lefthanders. Since a majority of the injured children would be righthanded, there will be very few cases in which handedness shifts as a result of right hemisphere lesions, but a large number in which it shifts as a result of left hemisphere lesions. Although this mechanism certainly must occur, it is questionable whether it could account for so large a percentage of twins of opposite handedness. Furthermore, it fails to account for the high rate of lefthandedness in first-degree relatives of twins. Boklage (1984) has pointed out that there is a 15% higher frequency of lefthandedness in second-born dizygotic twins than in their co-twins or siblings. This may well reflect birth trauma, but again it cannot account for the very high rate of lefthandedness in the first-degree relatives of twins.

Before discussing some possible causes of the dominance patterns of twins, let us consider some facts concerning multiple births. Monozygotic (identical) twins, who arise from the same fertilized egg, share the same chromosomes and therefore the same nuclear genes, whereas dizygotic (fraternal) twins, who are usually thought to result from the fertilization of two separate ova, are usually said to resemble each other on the average no more than any two siblings; that is, they share half their genes. Boklage (1984) believes that there may also be polar body twins. Before fertilization the ovum undergoes two divisions. In the first the number of chromosomes goes from the normal diploid number to the haploid number, in which each half carries half of the maternal chromosomes. The haploid ovum then undergoes division. One of the ova produced in the first division regresses to form the first polar body, which is then extruded. Similarly, in the second division one ovum regresses to form the second polar body. Boklage has suggested that in some cases the polar body does not regress and may also be fertilized by a different sperm. In this case the twins will be intermediate in genetic resemblance between dizygotic and monozygotic twins, sharing the same maternal chromosomes but, on the average, only half the paternal chromosomes. Polar body twins will thus share, on the average, three-quarters of their genes.

It is possible, however, that the genetic resemblance of both monozygotic twins and polar body twins may be less than these theoretical figures. Monozygotic twins are the result of cleavage of a fertilized ovum into two zygotes. The maternal genes carried in the cytoplasm of the ovum may be distributed unequally to the two zygotes. If cytoplasmic genes play a role in laterality, the offspring might differ. The same considerations apply, perhaps even more strongly, to polar body twins, since the division of the cytoplasm is so unequal.

The rate of monozygotic twinning is very much the same throughout the world: about 3 twin births per 1000. The dizygotic twinning rate, however, varies considerably. Thus, some older data showed that in Japan there was approximately 1 dizygotic twin birth out of 165, whereas in the northern countries of Ireland and Scotland the rate was about three times as high. The rates in northern Europe are generally of this order, and those in southern Europe are lower (Bulmer 1970). The highest twinning rates so far observed occur in West Africa, particularly among the Yoruba, especially in the vicinity of Ibadan, where the rate is about 1 in 18 births. In young Yoruba women of high parity the rate of twinning may be nearly 1 in 10 births. It is no surprise that twin dolls are a characteristic feature of Yoruba art. In the United States, Blacks (most of West African descent) have higher twinning rates, and Orientals have lower twinning rates than Caucasians (Bulmer 1970).

Familial monozygotic twinning is rare and does not share the high rate of congenital anomalies observed among familial dizygotic twins, which are much more common. Recent data from Italy (Parisi et al. 1983) suggest, however, that monozygotic twinning may occur more often than expected in families in which dizygotic twinning is found. There is also a high rate of neural tube defects in many populations in which dizygotic twinning is common, as it is in Ireland and Scotland. In China, where the rate of dizygotic twinning is very low, neural tube defects occur about one-tenth as frequently as in Ireland (Ghosh et al. 1981). It is very possible that the rate of twin conceptions is higher than is generally appreciated, since in some cases one fetus may die and be resorbed. The rate of twinning has been falling in recent years in Europe, as has the rate of neural tube defects, data for which no satisfactory explanation has yet been found.

The possible relationship between twinning and dominance may be revealed in part by considering some known influences on twinning. Mothers treated for infertility with either human chorionic gonadotropin or clomiphene have markedly increased rates of multiple births (Huppert 1979). Because of the high gonadotropin levels in both forms of therapy, more follicles mature and release ova, thus increasing the rate of dizygotic twinning. There are other circumstances in which gonadotropin levels can be high. Masculinized females, who by our hypothesis should have a high rate of personal and familial anomalous dominance, have elevated levels of luteinizing hormone (Jaffee and Vaitukaitis 1982). Since their offspring may have greater exposure to masculinizing effects in utero, they may have an elevated rate of lefthandedness. This hypothesis is compatible with the higher rate of lefthandedness in mothers of twins and in the twins themselves.

There are two other possible reasons for a higher rate of lefthandedness in twins. The first is that since the mothers will tend to be masculinized, they will often come from families with a tendency to greater testosterone production or sensitivity, and this will be shared by the twins. The second reason is essentially nongenetic. Since male twins both produce testosterone, each will conceivably be exposed to higher levels than he would be if he were a singleton. By this hypothesis, the females of opposite-sex pairs should have a high rate of lefthandedness, because of exposure to testosterone produced by the male co-twins. This type of effect has been observed in rats. A female rat lying in the uterus with males behind her will show a greater degree of androgen effects than other females, since the vasculature will carry testosterone from the males in an anterior direction (Meisel and Ward 1981). Other studies on the rat also document masculinizing effects by males on females in utero (Gandelman, vom Saal, and Reinisch 1977; Hauser and Gandelman 1983). The least testosterone effect should be found in all-female pairs. In all-male pairs one twin should be subject to a higher level of testosterone than the other. Glick (1983) has found that the rate of turning to the left in response to amphetamine is higher in female rats from litters with higher percentages of male siblings.

Another result in keeping with the hypothesis is the reported higher rate of dyslexia among twins (Bakwin 1973).

Further studies are suggested by these conjectures. Although masculinized women have a low fertility rate, one might expect them to show an elevated rate of twin births. One might also expect a higher rate of twin births among DES daughters.

Boklage observed an elevated rate of lefthandedness among the fathers, as well as among the mothers, of twins. This might occur because some of the sperm of lefthanded fathers have special properties; for example, they might be more likely to be successful in fertilizing ova, which would lead to a rise in dizygotic twinning. The zygotes resulting from fertilization might have a higher rate of cleavage into twin zygotes, which would favor monozygotic twinning. If the polar bodies of such zygotes regressed less often, polar body twinning would occur more frequently. We have already pointed out that the allele t associated with the major histocompatibility complex of the mouse does alter the behavior of sperm and is transmitted to offspring from fathers more frequently than the 50% expectation. If t-bearing sperm had an increased potential for fertilization of an ovum, then an elevated frequency of twins might be expected. If the same effect were found in the human, this would lead to an increased number of twin offspring. Since the T/t locus in the human has not been positively identified, it is conceivable that its behavior might be different. As already noted, the allele t in the mouse is associated with disorders similar to neural tube defects, so that it may play a role in formation of the central nervous system. We have already commented on the association of rates for twinning and neural tube disorders.

A relationship between sperm characteristics and lateralization is strongly suggested by the findings in Kartagener syndrome, in which affected males have situs inversus and sperm abnormalities (Afzelius et al. 1978). In patients with celiac disease, who have high rates of lefthandedness, sperm abnormalities are also common (Farthing et al. 1982). The possible relationships between sperm abnormalities and laterality determination will be discussed in chapter 19.

In any case the mechanism of the effect of paternal lefthandedness on twinning remains unclear. This problem too should be amenable to study in laboratory animals.

13.8 The Diversity of the Brain

There are critical periods for the development of structures during which they are particularly susceptible to external influences. For example, radiation will lead to an increased rate of cleft palate only during a particular, very short period. The existence of such critical periods is a useful strategy for reducing the possibilities of interference with normal development, since a rapidly developing structure will not be susceptible during most of pregnancy, and a deleterious effect manifest at some particular time will damage only a few structures. The development of the cortex does not appear to be an example of this mechanism, however, since it appears to continue through much of pregnancy and also during a significant period following birth. The cortex is presumably protected to a considerable extent by the presence of an excess of neurons during intrauterine life (and probably in the early postnatal period), which tends to guard against harmful effects of localized destruction at a particular time. This long period of development may confer benefits that outweigh the disadvantages of exposure to injury over an extended period. If a system is capable of being altered at many different periods by random influences occurring over a long time, then genetic determination of the final form will be much weaker than it is for systems that mature over a very brief span and are therefore less likely to be modified by outside agents. The genetic determination of lateralization will be weaker in the cortex than it is in other structures if even only a few of the nongenetic effects listed earlier are significant. The nervous system is subject to many influences that can alter the process at many times during pregnancy and postnatally. It has recently been pointed out that the appearance of long fiber tracts in the course of evolution makes the developing nervous system more subject to external influences, since the growth of such tracts necessarily requires a long period of time (McAllister et al. 1983).

The pattern of cortical development may well reflect a mechanism that is advantageous to the population as a whole, since it leads to a great diversity of patterns of lateralization, and therefore of patterns of talent. Since the cortex deals relatively little with elementary mechanisms immediately related to survival, the organism can tolerate a much greater degree of variation. This fact is probably reflected in different patterns of neuronal maturation. In some cases, as for example in the visual system and skeletal muscle, neurons appear to be directed to very precise targets. By contrast, the development of the cortex appears to allow for a higher rate of remodeling as cell death occurs. This diversity increases the probability that an unexpected problem can be met effectively by the cognitive specialization of some member of the population. This mechanism of diversity exacts a price, however, since the possibilities of interference over the long developmental period are great and the way is opened to unpleasant consequences such as childhood autism or dyslexia.

If these speculations are correct, one can be hopeful about possibilities of successful intervention, technically less elaborate possibilities than those required in a situation of more exact genetic determinism. The many routes of access to the system by environmental manipulation make possible relatively simple methods of modification without resort (except rarely) to more complex possibilities, such as genetic engineering. In theory it should be possible to specify which parents were more likely to have children with serious developmental disorders and to apply preventive measures. The more precisely the details of the processes are known, the more exactly one could in theory prevent deleterious effects without sacrificing the advantages of the diversity of the system. The great diversity of the nongenetic effects on lateralization probably explains most of the difficulties in setting up genetic theories of handedness.

13.9 Age and Ethnic Differences in Lateralization

Recent data suggest that the rate of nonrighthandedness is higher in the young, at least in Europe and the United States (Porac and Coren 1981; McGee and Cozad 1980). It is likely, for reasons we will not discuss, that this does not reflect a tendency for individuals to use the right hand more with increasing age but instead reflects declining pressures against the use of the left hand. It is important to keep these age-related differences in mind in research.

It is often assumed that the incidence of lefthandedness has varied little across history and across different ethnic populations. The available data suggest that in historical times lefthandedness has been present in some minority, ranging perhaps from 5% to 10% (Porac and Coren 1981). There is, however, no assurance that the rate of lefthandedness is not 30% or 50% higher now in certain populations than it was thousands of years ago. Furthermore, most of the current handedness data have been collected in the United States and in northern European and French-speaking populations. Very few studies have been conducted in Asia. One of these documented a lower rate of lefthandedness among children in Taiwan than is reported in the West (Teng, Lee, and Yang 1976). Another reported data on handedness in Japanese students, but, because of the tests used, it is not comparable to Western studies (Shimizu and Endo 1983). It is our impression, however, that extreme righthandedness was more common than in the West. It is sometimes asserted that dyslexia is less frequent among the Japanese and Chinese because of their ideographic scripts, but fully adequate data are not available. Perhaps the best test would be to study Japanese individuals attending English-speaking schools in the United States, since this would remove the questions raised by differences in the written language.

It is likely that, on the average, populations will differ in brain development, structure, and metabolism and therefore in lateralization patterns. Some brain diseases show marked ethnic variation; for example, Tay-Sachs disease and dystonia musculorum deformans occur predominantly in some Jewish populations. In northern Europe there is generally a higher frequency of twinning and of neural tube defects than in southern Europe and the Orient. Since twinning is associated with lefthandedness in whites, one might speculate that lefthandedness was less common in southern Europe and Japan and that therefore dyslexia and other learning disorders might be less frequent. There is a high rate of lefthandedness and of twinning in the parents of children with neural tube defects (Fraser, Czeizel, and Hanson 1982; LeMarec et al. 1978). This line of reasoning suggests that West Africa would have a very high rate of lefthandedness, learning disorders, and possibly neural tube defects, since this area has by far the highest reported twinning rates. There is evidence compatible with at least parts of this hypothesis. Stuttering is very common among schoolchildren in West Africa, the rates often being three times those found in the United States (Goodall and Brobby 1982). Blacks in the United States, mostly of West African origin, have higher stuttering rates than Caucasians. The hypothesis advanced to explain the West African data was the high prevalence of sickle-cell disease. An alternative interpretation is that in West Africa there is a high frequency of anomalous dominance and therefore of learning disorders, lefthandedness, and the other attendant talents and disabilities. The very few studies of handedness in Africa have shown very low apparent rates of lefthandedness, but it is not clear whether powerful cultural biases might be present.

The discussion of ethnic differences in handedness thus rests at present on mere fragments of information. It should be pointed out, however, that the distinctions so far presented are not between the conventional Caucasian, Black, and Oriental groups. Thus, the blond-haired, blue-eyed, and fair-skinned northern Europeans might resemble West African Blacks, whereas the Japanese might bear close resemblances to southern European Caucasians. We know of no available information on some of the largest groups, such as the Indian and Arab populations, although Indian twinning rates tend to be comparable to those found in Europe (Bulmer 1970). Similarly, East African populations could well differ from West African in the organization of laterality, just as they differ in so many other respects. It seems likely that very important information could be obtained by studying isolated populations such as those found in New Guinea or Australia or in other parts of Africa.

There are several reasons for studying populations that carry different genetic pools. For example, there is a very high risk of describing as universal human biology the properties of the best-studied populations, consisting to a very great extent of individuals of northern European descent. Moreover, differences between populations may cast important light on the mechanisms that produce lateralization and the disturbances that lead to learning disabilities. It is likely that studies of this type will ultimately benefit each group by providing information that will help to prevent or cure some of the brain disorders present in higher frequency in that population.

14　Disease Associations with Gender, Laterality, Dominance, and Learning Disabilities

Throughout this book we have repeatedly stressed selective unilateral developmental effects, hormonal atmosphere in pregnancy, the mechanisms of dominance, and the special association of learning disabilities with unilateral delays in development. Each of these factors may have special disease associations. The hormonal effects imply that many disorders might be related to gender. Certain diseases should show preferential involvement of one side of the brain or the body. The dominance pattern of an individual may be related to many disease susceptibilities, and the learning disorders group has several distinctive disease associations. We have already discussed conditions related to these factors. Here we wish to call attention specifically to this group of important factors that have often been overlooked in the past, and to awaken the interest of others in them.

The title of this chapter may suggest that what is to follow is a list of the disadvantages of individuals possessed of particular characteristics. We would again like to emphasize the frequent occurrence of advantages that often balance or even outweigh unfavorable susceptibilities. The special risk of females for many disorders is far outweighed by their lower rates of coronary disease and lung cancer. It is likely that the same is true for all other groups. Whether a group is at net advantage or disadvantage can be ascertained only by knowing the rates of all causes of morbidity and mortality.

Although many of the disease associations of these factors are undoubtedly related to the mechanisms we have discussed, we are, of course, aware that many other factors may be at work.

14.1 Diseases with Unilateral Predominance

The possibility of unilateral predominance is often overlooked, although data exist for certain conditions. Disorders of any of the unpaired organs are necessarily asymmetrical, but many disorders, even in paired organs, affect one side preferentially (Schnall and Smith 1974).

Undescended testes are located significantly more often on the right side, although the effect is not large. In a Chinese study the right testis was higher and heavier than the left in most cases (Chang et al. 1960). The right testis develops earlier than the left, just as the left ovary precedes the right (Mittwoch 1975). In hermaphrodites who have an ovary and a testis, the latter is usually on the right, presumably because it develops earlier than the ovary.

Cancers and cysts of the breast are found to a small but significant extent more frequently on the right than on the left. The same has been reported for supernumerary nipples, breast hypertrophy, and difficulties in lactation (Howard et al. 1982).

The curious condition of hemihypertrophy (Poskanser 1975; Gesell 1927) deserves comment. In this disorder one entire side of the body is larger than the other, although in rare cases there is hypertrophy of the upper limbs on one side and the lower on the other. The patients have high rates of mental defects and neoplasms, such as Wilms's tumor. Neoplasms occur with higher frequency on the involved side, which may have a higher skin temperature; there may be more rapid growth in tissue culture of fibroblasts from the larger side. Some series suggest a right-sided predominance. Hemiatrophy appears in isolation or as a component of Russel-Silver syndrome and is more frequent on the left side (Schnall and Smith 1974). Many other unilateral conditions, such as the preferentially left-sided location of papillomas of the choroid plexus and intraventricular meningiomas, will be discussed in other sections.

14.2 Gender-related Disease Susceptibility

The statement that disease associations with laterality, gender, dominance, and learning disabilities have been neglected might appear at least in part to be incorrect. In any textbook of medicine gender is by far the most commonly mentioned risk factor. Even a brief inspection will show the correctness of this statement. Among the major killers cardiovascular disease, cancer of the lung, and cancer of the colon are male predominant, whereas cancer of the breast occurs only rarely in men. Hemochromatosis is strongly male predominant. Photosensitive porphyria is more frequent in males, though the opposite is true for the acute intermittent form. Although examples could readily be multiplied, our point remains valid since the reasons for the male-female differences are rarely discussed, although they must be of great importance. Some are nonhormonal; such factors especially affecting men include cigarette smoking, alcoholism, occupational exposure, and dietary habits. Other differences must relate to adult hormonal factors. Still others, we believe, must be produced by intrauterine or early postnatal hormone effects; in these cases dominance, laterality, and learning disorder associations should also be common.

Gender susceptibility transcends spontaneous disease. There are very large differences between males and females in susceptibility to many drugs and toxins (Selye 1971), yet these are generally neglected in pharmacology texts and tend to be overlooked in discussions of drug therapy and its complications. Many of the gender differences in immunity, metabolism, and drug responsiveness are established in the intrauterine or early postnatal developmental period and are often not reversible at later ages by the administration of hormones. Some of these metabolic forms of imprinting will be discussed in a later section.

Administration of the appropriate hormone during a critical period can in some cases induce the pattern of responsiveness to drugs or toxins typical of one gender group in individuals of the other group. Rat females exposed early to testosterone will permanently show a pattern of testosterone responsiveness similar to that of males. The pattern of sex hormones in adult life may, however, in some cases mask or alter certain susceptibilities determined in utero. We have proposed that the heightened susceptibility to certain immune diseases in those with anomalous dominance is the result of effects on the developing immune system of a male-related factor. Yet adult onset immune disorders are in general less frequent in males than in females; we have hypothesized that this might be due to a protective effect of the postpubertal rise of testosterone. There must be many other examples of modification by later hormonal environment of the susceptibilities set in utero.

14.3 Relationships of Cerebral Dominance to Disease

The higher rates of immune disorders and migraine in lefthanders have already been mentioned. Parenthetically, we should note that migraine is related to all of the factors discussed: unilateral predilection, female predominance, and an association with lefthandedness and learning disorders. The older literature contains references to associations of handedness with somatic disease, learning disorders, and psychiatric disorders; many of these are discussed in other sections.

14.4 Disease Associations and Developmental Disorders

Several authors have described an elevated frequency of certain diseases in children with learning disorders. One of our hypotheses is that many of the associations of learning disorders are more generally associations of anomalous dominance. It is easy to understand the earlier emphasis on the association with learning disorders rather than with lefthandedness or anomalous dominance. Since children with learning disorders are often collected in special clinics or institutions, the other medical conditions present in these patients may more easily come to the attention of physicians.

We believe that the majority, and possibly nearly all, children with learning disorders are drawn from the anomalous dominance population. The question must arise whether those with learning disorders are more often subject to these diseases than are those with anomalous dominance but without learning disorders. Within the group with learning disorders, one might expect degrees of anomalous dominance, perhaps with corresponding variations in disease associations. M. Kinsbourne and B. Bemporad (personal communication) found a higher rate of immune disease in the families of dyslexics who were lefthanded or had lefthanded relatives than in the families of dyslexics without such histories.

We must also ask whether the elevated susceptibility to certain immune disorders among those with anomalous dominance is associated with a changed susceptibility to infection—for example, a decreased risk of acquiring certain infections but an increased risk of acquiring others. We will return to the question of infection in chapter 16.

14.4.1 Vestibular and Eye Movement Disorders

The literature on learning disorders contains many papers dealing with alterations in the vestibular system and in eye movement (Pirozzolo and Hansch 1982). Some have even attempted to link the mechanisms of learning disorders and schizophrenia to these associated anomalies. We suspect, however, that vestibular and oculomotor anomalies in learning disorders and in some psychiatric conditions do not play a role in causing the deviant behavior but are instead parallel effects of the causes of these behavioral disorders. Vestibular anomalies may derive from lateral imbalances produced in normally symmetrical neural systems by alterations in hemispheric dominance relationships. It is often stated that there is a high frequency of childhood motion sickness among those with learning disorders, but this has not been documented. A past or current history of motion sickness is common in migraine (Barbas, Matthews, and Ferrari 1983; Kuritzky, Ziegler, and Hassanein 1981), a condition associated with a higher frequency of lefthandedness than is present in the general population. An anomalous vestibular system may well be present in torsion dystonia and spasmodic torticollis (Stejskal and Tomanek 1981), since the direction of head turning in any affected individual corresponds to the direction in which induced nystagmus tends to be greatest. This report denied any relationship to the handedness of the subjects, but since only five subjects were lefthanded, further studies are warranted.

Several mechanisms might lead to an elevated rate of vestibular anomalies in subjects with anomalous dominance. One such mechanism might be abnormalities in the formation of the vestibular systems in the brainstem. Another speculative possibility would tie vestibular changes to altered cortical mechanisms. Some authors have suggested that there is a cortical representation of the vestibular system in the temporal lobe in close proximity to the cortical auditory systems (Crosby, Humphrey, and Lauer 1962). In primates lesions of this cortex can lead to dramatic spontaneous rotation. Temporal lobe epilepsy occasionally produces powerful sensations of rotation that can mimic attacks of acute vestibular dysfunction. This type of sensation would arise from the superior portions of the temporal lobe if the human vestibular cortex were comparable to that of the monkey. Anomalies of development in or near this location should, however, not be rare, since the cytoarchitectonic defects in dyslexics appear to have a predilection for this late-developing region of the temporal lobe.

Several types of disturbance might result from abnormal formation of the cortex in this region (for example, seizures with an aura of vertigo, which do occur, although uncommonly). In some cases a spike focus in this location might lead either to a distortion of the stimuli reaching the vestibular cortex or to distortion of the response pattern. Even in the absence of abnormal electrical activity anomalous formation of this region might lead to altered responses to vestibular inputs. One might speculate that the normal vestibular system is balanced (that is, there is little bias in either direction), so that stimuli in one direction will on the average be balanced by stimuli in the other direction. Anomalous formation of the vestibular cortex might disturb this balance, thus favoring motion sickness and also a greater bias for eye movements to one side. Although speculative, these considerations are amenable to experimental study. The existence of a bias of the kind suggested might also play a role in such conditions as spasmodic torticollis.

14.4.2 Mirror Reading, Mirror Writing, and Mirror Movements

Orton (1925) pointed out that some childhood dyslexics could read better in a mirror or with a book held upside down (in which case the print is both inverted and reversed). There has been a marked revival of interest in this phenomenon. One hypothesis is that reading is hampered in these patients when eye movements are not in a preferred direction, but there is at least one other possible explanation. In the normal reading of languages such as English, written from left to right, the next words to be read lie to the right of the fixation point (that is, in the right visual field); they are, therefore, projected to the *left* hemisphere. When words are presented in mirror fashion, the next words to be read reach the right hemisphere. If the left hemisphere is less efficient than the right in processing visual language, reading might be more adequate if the message could reach the right side of the brain. It might be argued that if the left hemisphere systems were inadequate, the callosal projections would simply relay the visual language message to the more competent right side. The anomalous development of the cortex on the left might, however, also lead to disturbance of callosal projections, which originate partly in cortex. (We will return to the issue of the anomalous callosal projections in chapter 15.) A possible explanation of superior reading of words presented in mirror fashion is, therefore, that the message is transmitted to the more efficient reading-related areas of the right hemisphere; when words are presented in the standard left-to-right fashion, they fail to be transmitted to the right hemisphere because the necessary callosal connections are poorly formed in many dyslexics.

P. Udden (personal communication) has suggested that those dyslexics who find it easier to read English in mirror fashion might not have been dyslexic in learning to read Hebrew, which is written in the reverse direction. This raises the possibility that a different group of individuals would be dyslexic in Hebrew, namely, those who have superior reading ability in the left hemisphere. This group would prefer to read Hebrew in mirror fashion. We suspect, however, that those dyslexics who read English better in mirror fashion would still be dyslexic in Hebrew, although probably less so, because even when the right hemisphere has superior capacities for reading, it is probably not as competent as a normal left hemisphere. On the other hand, the great bulk of Israelis who have a left hemisphere with superior capacities for reading will not be dyslexic in learning to read Hebrew. Although the written word will typically be projected to the right hemisphere, their normal callosal connections will relay the message to the more efficient left hemisphere. Since our belief is that those dyslexic in learning Hebrew would be drawn from the same population, they too would have an elevated rate of nonrighthandedness. Udden has suggested to us that the same mechanism might account for the preference of some lefthanders to write with a hooked position or, in the extreme case, in mirror fashion—that is, in such a manner as to make the words more easily read by the right hemisphere. The notebooks of Leonardo da Vinci, who was lefthanded, were written in inverted and reversed fashion. A finding compatible with this hypothesis is that in Israel lefthanders write much less frequently in the hooked position (Moscovitch and Smith 1979). The ability to read and write in mirror fashion is much more common in lefthanders. A few nonrighthanders can even write one sentence forward with one hand and a different sentence in mirror fashion with the other. It was said of President James Garfield, who was lefthanded, that he could in fact do this in two different languages. (There is a hint that Garfield was mathematically inclined, since he devised a proof of the Pythagorean theorem.) These findings suggest not only bilateral representation of language and pyramidal motor control but also a lack of interference effects between the two sides as the result of a defect in callosal connectivity.

The hooked writing position is seen in many lefthanders, particularly males. Although this is a fascinating and complex phenomenon, we will not explore it in detail. The studies of Levy and Reid who originally drew attention to it (Levy and Reid 1976), suggest anomalous connectivity in this group. This raises the important possibility that there are multiple forms of nonrighthandedness, varying according to the particular motor systems involved.

Mirror movements (the involuntary movements of one side upon voluntary movements of the other) represent a disturbance of laterality, of which the mechanism has not yet been worked out. There is a general belief that these movements are also more common in nonrighthanders, and this fits in with our experience. Although marked degrees of mirror movement will often attract attention, our experience suggests that minor degrees of this disturbance are more common than is generally appreciated. We have also seen individuals with anomalous dominance in whom mirror movements are present at certain times and absent at others. Two such patients with anomalous dominance had an intermittent tremor, accompanied by mirror movements that disappeared when the tremor improved. This may suggest participation of subcortical motor mechanisms in mirror movements. It would be of interest to know whether propranolol would diminish some forms of mirror movement.

Congenital mirror movements, which may appear in families, are sometimes so severe as to be disabling. An odd association is the frequent presence of Klippel-Feil syndrome and other bony anomalies of the cervical spine in such patients (Regli, Filippa, and Wiesendanger 1967). This has suggested the likelihood of an associated anomaly in the adjacent region of the junction of the spinal cord and medulla, very possibly in the decussation of the pyramidal tracts. One group has argued for cortical anomalies in these cases (Harati, Meyer, and Wheeler 1981). It is possible that more than one mechanism causes mirror movements and also that affected individuals have several related anomalies. Woods and Eby (1982) have found that mentally defective children with mirror movements are more aggressive on the average than those without them.

Acquired mirror movements may throw some light on this problem. We believe, however, that not all acquired mirror movements have the same mechanism. Thus, in acquired hemiplegia (Woods and Teuber 1978) mirror movements tend to occur in the *intact* hand on the attempt to move the paretic one. Our guess is that this does not reflect a release in involuntary mirror movements. One possibility is that, as a result of damage to the motor systems of one hemisphere, the patient attempts to use bilaterally distributed motor systems from the other hemisphere. Mirror movements are occasionally seen on the paretic side with movements of the intact one, which presumably have a different mechanism. In unilaterally predominant parkinsonism we have several times seen mirror movements in the *affected* limb on movement of the less involved side.

A progressive syndrome has been described in three patients of Irish descent, which began with involvement of the left limbs (Rebeiz, Kolodny, and Richardson 1968). Pyramidal, basal ganglia, and cerebellar signs can be observed. One patient seen by us displayed dramatic mirror movements involving the entire affected left arm when the right arm moved.

No study has yet been made of anomalous dominance in relation to acquired mirror movements, a topic that deserves study.

15

Asymmetries in the
Neural Crest and
Other Systems

In the preceding chapters we have developed the hypothesis that variations in asymmetry of neurological function reflect influences, often of an endocrine or immune nature, acting during the development of the nervous system. We believe that patterns of development of other organs may also be altered along with the structures underlying dominance.

Most of the subsequent chapters will be devoted to these implications. In certain cases we believe that reasonable evidence already exists for some of the links suggested; in other cases the discussion will center on topics that can be elucidated only by further study. We believe it is important to present these more speculative possibilities, which suggest fruitful areas of research.

15.1 Asymmetry in the Neural Crest

In this section we will discuss the possibility of asymmetry in development of derivatives of the neural crest, a possibility suggested to us both by personal clinical observations and by findings in the literature.

The neural crest is a particularly interesting structure that develops on the lips of the neural tube (LeDouarin 1982). It is therefore not surprising that it plays a major role in the formation of the nervous system, giving rise to all the dorsal root ganglia as well as to autonomic ganglia and several of the ganglia of the cranial nerves. It also forms both leptomeninges and dura in the forebrain (though not in the hindbrain or spinal cord). Its participation in the formation of nonneural tissues is equally extensive. Nearly every pigmented cell of the body originates in the crest, a point of major importance, since so many anomalies of neural crest origin, in whatever tissue they are located, may be accompanied by changes in skin pigmentation (such as hyperpigmented or hypopigmented areas) or of other structures within the skin (such as vascular nevi).

Derivatives of the neural crest form several other tissues. Of special interest are the connective tissue of the thymus gland (the epithelium that processes lymphocytes being of different origin) and the skin and bones of the face (LeDouarin 1982). The importance of this structure actually extends to many other tissues, which it does not form directly. In Di George syndrome, in which several crest derivatives fail to develop, the thymus either is undeveloped or fails to develop altogether. The absence of the crest-derived thymic connective tissue leads to a lack of the inductive influence necessary for formation of the epithelium. Similarly, tooth development can be impaired. Lesions of the cephalic neural crest have been found to lead to lack of development, or underdevelopment, of the thymus and the thyroid, along with cardiac lesions (Bockman and Kirby 1984).

Disorders of crest development may have even more profound effects on the nervous system. The Siamese cat, which is an albino, has an anomalous pattern of decussation of the optic nerves, which is probably the result of lack of melanin-bearing cells in the pigment epithelium of the retina. Recent work supports the view that melanin-bearing cells may be necessary to act as guides for migrating optic nerve fibers (Strongin and Guillery 1981; Witkop et al. 1982). If the same is true elsewhere, failures of neural crest formation or migration may underlie anomalous neural pathway formation in other regions. It would therefore not be surprising if an elevated rate of disordered neural crest derivatives were to be found in the anomalous dominance population. The pigmented cells of the retina are not of neural crest origin (LeDouarin 1982). It remains to be shown that pigmented cells elsewhere play a role in migration of axons. Certain suggestive data do exist, however. For example, light hair is more common in harelip patients than in the unaffected (Tisserand 1949). Neural tube defects such as spina bifida are many times more common in the northern British Isles than in the Orient (Ghosh et al. 1981), and in the United States they are more common in Caucasian than Black infants.

Indirect evidence exists that sex hormones play a role in crest development, although this has to our knowledge not yet been studied directly. Melanomas are known in some instances to carry estradiol receptors, and they have sometimes been treated with the estrogen antagonist tamoxifen. Intracranial meningiomas may carry estradiol receptors, and, as noted, the meninges of the forebrain are crest derivatives. The recently described association of meningiomas with breast cancer raises the possibility that some common endocrinological factor is operative in intrauterine life. In any case the possibility should be considered that hormonal effects on neuronal migration might be accompanied by alterations in crest derivatives. Another possibly relevant fact is that neurofibromatosis, which appears to be predominantly a neural crest disorder, typically worsens at puberty, particularly in females, and in pregnancy. Since adrenal steroids are known to affect certain aspects of neural crest development, it would not be surprising if sex steroids also played a role.

Meningiomas of the lateral ventricle are much more common on the left, and this raises the possibility of asymmetry in neural crest migrations. Conceivably, certain delaying influences produce parallel unilateral effects on both neural tube and neural crest derivatives. Another possibility is that some of the delaying factors act primarily on the left neural crest and thus secondarily lead to failures in neuronal or axonal migration.

15.1.1 Cardiac Asymmetry and Congenital Anomalies

There are nonneural sites in which the neural crest may well play a role in asymmetry. The connective tissue and muscular walls of the great vessels arising from the aortic arch are of neural crest origin (LeDouarin 1982). Interference with the embryonic neural crest leads to anomalies at this site (Bockman and Kirby 1984), including transposition of the great vessels, a disorder that, along with congenital heart block, has been described in the children of female patients with lupus erythematosus (Esscher and Scott 1979; Vetter and Raskind 1983). In preliminary studies we have found a high rate of both of these anomalies in the families of dyslexics (P. Behan and N. Geschwind, personal observations).

15.1.2 Harelip, Cleft Palate, and Anomalies of the Face and Ears

There are several other examples of asymmetrical formation of neural crest derivatives. The skin and bones of the face and part of the skull (but not in other regions) derive from the neural crest, and harelip is now regarded as a neural crest disturbance (LeDouarin 1982). Two-thirds of all harelips lie on the left side. Of 200 patients with harelip

20% were lefthanded versus 8% of 200 controls (Tisserand 1944). Righthanded patients with harelip had twice as high a number of lefthanded relatives as unaffected righthanders. Another relationship to the neural crest may be reflected in the later finding that dark hair was found in only about 6% of individuals with harelip but in 28% of controls.

The data on harelip reveal one odd feature. Despite Tisserand's (1944) finding that two-thirds of all harelips lay on the left, the rate of left-sided involvement was about 50% in the lefthanded and about 70% in the righthanded, a difference that is statistically significant. Put in another form, of those with right harelip 30% are lefthanded, and of those with left harelip 15% are lefthanded. More information is needed concerning details of the times when the anlage of the lip is being formed in relation to when the neural areas that control handedness are being laid down. The possibility must also be considered that the fetal death rate is higher among those with left harelip and left dominance. It is, however, also possible that these apparently paradoxical data reflect the use of the dichotomous categories of right and lefthandedness. The majority of the harelip patients either were lefthanded or had first-degree lefthanded relatives. It is quite possible that most of the so-called righthanders among the left-sided harelip patients were actually individuals who on a handedness battery would have had scores in the intermediate ranges. If this were true, then there could have been a higher percentage of nonrighthanders in the left-sided than in the right-sided harelip group.

In the rat adrenal steroids given at the proper time in pregnancy lead to a high rate of cleft palate in the offspring. We are not familiar with similar studies on the effects of gonadal steroids. There is a high rate of epilepsy among the parents of cleft palate and harelip patients, and anticonvulsant treatment has been suggested as a likely cause of some of the cases. Other data suggest that the rate of harelip and cleft palate may be elevated even in the absence of such treatment. These findings suggest that disorders of neuronal migration accompany disturbed migration in the neural crest.

Many syndromes are associated with unusual facial features. Malformed or malpositioned ears are commonly seen. The extreme example of low-set ears is otocephaly, which is also a neural crest anomaly (LeDouarin 1982). Asymmetry of the external ear canals occurs in less than 30% of the normal population but is present in over 65% of the mentally retarded and learning disabled (Durfee 1974).

Such anomalies may well be expected to be more common in the anomalous dominance population. There are individuals with markedly asymmetrical facial size, which we have seen several times in association with scoliosis. The extreme case, facial hypoplasia (Aase and Smith 1970), is more common on the left side. Since this is probably also a neural crest anomaly, it provides further evidence for asymmetry of neural crest migrations. In particular, it suggests that these migrations are more likely to be delayed on the left, just like those in the cortex.

15.1.3 Scoliosis

Another condition in which neural crest migration may play a role is scoliosis. We cannot review all the theories concerning this disorder, but we will discuss one particular group of studies. In the young experimental animal dorsal root destruction is often effective in producing scoliosis (Liszka 1961; MacEwen 1972; Alexander, Bunch, and Ebbesson 1972). One possibility is that spinal curvature is induced by the asymmetrical proprioceptive input, which the animal responds to as if the spine were being bent to one side. Another mechanism is suggested by the finding that removal of dorsal root ganglia in the developing frog leads to a reduction in motoneurons in the corresponding segments and possibly to an increased number in adjacent segments (Davis, Constantine-Paton, and Schorr 1983). The authors cite another study in which it was found that early neural crest removal in the chick reduced motoneuron populations. Alexander, Bunch, and Ebbesson (1972) found that dorsal rhizotomy led to scoliosis only when the anterior horn cell changes were produced.

We are indebted to Dr. Melvin Glimcher, Professor of Orthopedics at the Harvard Medical School, an outstanding authority on bone, for some comments on this mechanism. He points out that the procedure of cutting posterior roots does not lead to scoliosis as reliably as removal of multiple ribs on one side. The latter procedure may not correspond to the causative mechanism in many cases of clinical scoliosis, however, since absence of ribs is surely a rare accompaniment of this disorder. We will present evidence that, by contrast, scoliosis is often found in clinical situations in which there is clear evidence of alteration of sensory systems, or of anomalies of the neural crest.

If this mechanism is responsible for some, and perhaps many, cases, one can envision that defective unilateral formation of the dorsal root ganglia, which are neural crest derivatives, might lead to scoliosis. This possibility is suggested by the clinical picture of a patient with scoliosis seen by one of us. He had total loss of all modalities of sensation from the nipple to the knee on one side with absent cremasteric and abdominal reflexes on that side. He also suffered from irregular skin pigmentation. This case raises the possibility that there was inadequate formation of dorsal root ganglia and pigmented cells on one side. Another patient was born with a hairy black nevus on one side of the lumbar spine and suffered from scoliosis. In later years he developed marked vitiligo, an immune disorder of melanocytes. Still later he was found to have a left frontal convexity meningioma. Two other patients of ours with meningiomas had nevi on the face or scalp.

Scoliosis is strongly associated with many hereditary or congenital neurological disorders affecting sensory systems in the spinal cord, such as the spinocerebellar ataxias, syringomyelia, and spinal gliomas. Scoliosis may accompany familial dysautonomia, in which there is deficit of neural crest derivatives (dorsal root autonomic ganglia). Furthermore, a special type of scoliosis is seen in neurofibromatosis, which, with its involvement of pigmented cells and Schwann cells (both neural crest derivatives), appears to be a neural crest disorder. In addition, there may be lack of bone in the wall of the orbit, also a neural crest derivative. Dr. Glimcher informs us that the scoliosis in this condition is distinctive in its pattern of involvement of a delimited number of spinal column segments. In any case this disorder again illustrates the association of scoliosis with a disorder of sensory systems and clear neural crest involvement. MacEwen (1972) found scoliosis in 20% of patients with cerebral palsy but did not discuss the presence of distinctive clinical features in this group.

A particularly intriguing feature of scoliosis is its relationship to sex and age. The largest group of patients, consisting of females in whom the major (thoracic) curve is typically convex to the left, often worsens at puberty. It is possible that this form of scoliosis is equally common in males but that it progresses much less often after puberty and therefore does not come to medical attention. The typical worsening after puberty, especially in females, strongly suggests a role of sex hormones. By contrast, in infantile scoliosis, a much rarer condition, males predominate and the major curve is in the opposite direction, convex to the right (Ponseti et al. 1976; Wynne-Davies 1978). In all of these infantile cases there is also underdevelopment of the face on the side of the convexity.

The asymmetry of scoliosis is suggestive of unilateral failure of dorsal root formation and therefore of unilateral disordered neural crest migrations. Further experimental studies will be required to verify the importance of this process in humans and to work out the details. It will obviously be important to study the handedness distribution in scoliosis of both types. It is our impression that the common later form of scoliosis is associated with an elevated rate of nonrighthandedness.

Scoliosis is very common among patients with spinal arachnoid cysts (Cilluffo et al. 1981). As we shall point out later, cysts of this type may well be caused in many cases by immune attack.

15.1.4 Pigmented Cells of Skin and Hair

If pigmented cells play an important role as guides to development of neural (and possibly other) structures, hypopigmented or irregularly pigmented individuals might be more susceptible to influences affecting migration and assembly of nerve cells and fibers. The Siamese cat, with its anomalous visual pathways and strabismus, is an example. The same types of effects might perhaps be expected among humans with light hair or eyes. In one study refraction defects were reported more commonly in those with light coloration, but strabismus was not discussed (Mieses-Reif 1936). It has been stated that lefthandedness is more common in strabismic patients, and Dr. Simmons Lessell in Boston has completed a study showing increased nonrighthandedness in patients with esotropia (crossed eyes) (personal communication). As mentioned earlier, Tisserand (1949) found that dark hair was much less common among harelip patients (who also have an excess of lefthandedness) than among controls. Studies are now underway to investigate these possibilities. We have found that blonds are significantly more nonrighthanded than brunettes (Schachter and Galaburda, in press). Thus, of 986 nonblonds 76% scored more than +70 on a modified Oldfield Handedness Battery (strongly righthanded), 12% scored in the 0 to +70 range (ambidextrous), and 12% scored in the 0–100 range (lefthanded). The corresponding figures for 131 blonds were 56%, 28%, and 16%; the difference in the distribution of scores in the two groups was highly significant.

It is our impression, though this has not yet been confirmed, that pigmentary anomalies are more common among individuals with anomalous dominance. Several such individuals we have seen have had facial nevi, either pigmented or vascular. The occurrence of vascular nevi at the same dermatomal level as a spinal vascular malformation was pointed out by Cobb (1915). Cushing (1906) had commented on a similar relationship between facial or scalp nevi and intracerebral vascular malformations. As noted earlier, we have now seen several patients with meningiomas who also had nevi; these were usually found on the face or scalp, though one patient had a black hairy nevus at the base of the spine. We have also seen patients with epilepsy with a facial nevus on the same side as the epileptic focus. The most dramatic example of a disorder of this type is Sturge-Weber syndrome, which in addition primarily affects females. It would be important to ascertain whether this affects predominantly one side.

Another important pigmentary anomaly is early gray or white hair. It is frequently stated in the lay literature that early gray or white hair is common in the families of dyslexics. It has been our impression that in fact early gray hair is more common among individuals with anomalous dominance and their relatives, which would include those with childhood learning disorders.

Early gray or white hair is of particular interest because of its known association with certain autoimmune diseases, the ones most often noted being pernicious anemia (Minot 1948) and autoimmune thyroid disorder (Wood 1983). In fact, we believe that it is even more widely associated with immune diseases. The association suggests immune attack on pigment cells in the hair follicles. Wood (1983) has confirmed the presence of a high rate of nonrighthandedness in patients with immune thyroid disease; he also found a high rate of early gray or white hair but did not report whether this was present more often in the lefthanded patients. An elevated rate of dyslexia was not found in the immune thyroid patients, but the series was probably too small to ascertain this point.

Certain other features associated with early gray hair deserve mention. Early graying has important ethnic associations, being more common among northern Europeans and, we suspect, Blacks of West African descent but less common among southern Europeans and Far Eastern populations. This deserves further study, since it would be in keeping with the possibility that anomalous dominance may be more common among northern Europeans and West Africans. In addition, the Japanese usually have sparse facial hair, and early baldness is less common among them than among northern Europeans. This suggests end-organ insensitivity of the hair follicles to dihydrotestosterone, but it is not clear whether this is related to the low prevalence of early gray or white hair.

We have observed another striking feature of those with early gray or white hair, namely, that affected males have a low rate of early male pattern baldness (which is very comon in populations of northern European descent) and that affected females tend to show thinning of the hair much less often after the menopause. Male pattern baldness and postmenopausal hair thinning occur only in the presence of androgens. The male with early white or gray hair is not usually hypogonadal or insensitive to androgens. Diminished hair loss therefore suggests low *local* sensitivity of the hair follicles to androgens. As noted earlier, testosterone in many instances protects from immune attack. The converse may also be true: immune attack on the pigmented cells of the hair follicles may lead to reduced sensitivity to androgenic effects. One possibility, though a speculative one, is that antibodies binding to the hair follicles present a barrier to androgens. We have noted the lower rate of early male pattern baldness and sparse facial hair among the Japanese, resulting from insensitivity of the hair follicles to dihydrotestosterone. It would be interesting to know whether Europeans or Blacks with early gray hair also need to shave less frequently—that is, whether the immune protection against androgens also extends to facial hair.

Eye color (the color of the iris) is another interesting feature. The Siamese cat, which is an albino, has a high rate of strabismus. Some older papers claimed, but without adequate documentation, that left-handedness was more frequent in those with strabismus. We have cited the as yet unpublished findings of Lessell supporting this claim. Korein (1981) reported that patients with dystonia and spasmodic torticollis displayed an elevated rate of blue or hazel eyes. Lang et al. (1982) disputed this, but Korein (1982) has pointed out that their data actually confirm his conclusions, a view with which we agree. We have also been interested in anomalies of iris pigmentation; for example, we have examined one woman (the mother of three lefthanded children) who has blue eyes, except that her left iris has one spoke of brown pigment. Another woman (the mother of a son with anomalous dominance) has one blue and one brown eye. This condition, called *heterochromia iridis*, is usually thought to result either from genetic mosaicism or from damage at birth to the superior cervical ganglion on one side. Since this can occur as a familial anomaly (Dahlberg 1944–47), it is likely that it can also result from delayed neural crest migration on one side.

Another intriguing phenomenon is asymmetrical loss of hair pigment. The most common example is the white forelock seen both in normals and in patients suffering from certain disorders such as Waardenburg syndrome; we know of no data on the relationship between this condition and lateral predominance or handedness. Even more common is asymmetrical frontal graying, with a sharp division at the midline, most readily observed in those with short curly hair. The possible relationships between such graying and cerebral laterality or lesions have not yet been investigated. An interesting possible example is a male patient in his sixties who suffered a spontaneous intracerebral hemorrhage from a very large aneurysm in the right anterior Sylvian fissure. His hair was short, tightly curled, and originally black in color. He had a striking pattern of graying, the right anterior frontal region of his hair being visibly much grayer than the left.

Rats treated in early life with cortisone, even if from an albino strain, are typically small and dark, showing that steroids can lead to lifting of the repression of the melanin-producing enzymes, which is present in many forms of albinism. These cortisone-treated animals are immunologically different from others of the same strain. In Addison's disease, with its low rate of adrenal steroid production, the skin also becomes darker. In any case we believe that skin pigmentation and iris pigmentation both reflect immunological, endocrinological, and dominance characteristics.

We will comment in section 16.1 on the remarkable phenomenon of new local changes in hair color at sites corresponding to a brain lesion.

15.1.5 Neurons of the Gut

It is also intriguing that the intrinsic neurons of the gut are of neural crest origin, in view of the especially high rate of gut-related immune disorders found in our studies of strong lefthanders. In the rat adrenal steroids increase the amount of catecholamine production in the enteric neurons and may also lead to anomalous placement of cells. It would be interesting to know about the effects of sex steroids.

15.2 Skeletal Anomalies and Neural Tube Defects

In addition to its association with the conditions already mentioned, we believe that anomalous dominance is associated in elevated frequency with disorders in other systems. At the time of the Geschwind and Behan study (1982) a surprising number of lefthanders added the notation to the questionnaire that they had situs inversus, but this remains to be studied formally. Alterations in the skeleton may be very common; we have already referred to scoliosis. It should be noted that in most people the right arm is longer than the left but the left foot is larger than the right; there are corresponding differences in muscle weight (Chhibber and Singh 1970, 1972). Even in utero the bones of the right arm and left leg are heavier than their opposites (Pande and Singh 1971). Curiously enough, the same pattern is found in the frog and the rabbit (Singh 1971). It may seem odd that the left leg is the larger, but it is reasonable teleologically at least in the human. If someone is rightfooted (for example, kicks with the right foot), the left leg will be used for bearing weight. In quadrupedal animals this advantage would not appear to be important. On the other hand, it might be related to the typical crossed pattern of locomotion; but it would be difficult to use this to explain the pattern in the frog.

It has been shown that the rate of lefthandedness is elevated in Legg-Perthe's disease (Burwell et al. 1978), which is male predominant. Dr. Melvin Glimcher has reviewed his own cases of this condition and finds a very high rate of lefthandedness, particularly among female patients. It is our impression that anomalies of the vertebral column (for instance Klippel-Feil syndrome and related disorders, and pilonidal sinus) are found in raised frequency in the anomalous dominance population. Furthermore, we believe that these skeletal anomalies are associated with a high rate of immune disease, but this remains to be documented. Since many of these anomalies of the vertebral column may reflect delayed closure of the neural tube, it is possible that the influences that produce them also lead to delayed formation of the left hemisphere and to slowing of immune development. One might therefore expect spina bifida and related disorders to have similar associations. Neural tube defects are in general more common in populations with high rates of twinning, a condition associated with an elevated rate of lefthandedness. In fact, there is a high rate of twinning among the parents of children with spina bifida

(LeMarec et al. 1978). Fraser (1983) has also found a high rate of lefthandedness in families of children with spina bifida.

The fact that neural tube defects are female predominant suggests a role for hormones. The very low rate of concordance for neural tube defects between identical twins strongly suggests a special role for environmental factors in pregnancy. Nance (1969) has brought evidence that neural tube defects are transmitted primarily from mothers. This might suggest cytoplasmic inheritance, but cytoplasmic inheritance alone would account neither for female predominance nor for low concordance between identical twins. Another possibility is that this condition reflects the action of maternal environmental influences on a genetically susceptible offspring. Some of these influences may be hormonal, possibly reflecting anomalous maternal hormone production. Neural tube defects may also have an immunological component, since a high rate of HLA concordance has been reported between the mothers and fathers of children with neural tube defects (Taylor and Faulk 1981; Faulk 1981). Even in this case hormonal effects may contribute; for example, in the presence of HLA concordance an anomalous hormonal atmosphere may markedly enhance the probability of neural tube defects. A role for the neural crest is suggested by the markedly higher rate of spina bifida in northern Britain than in the Orient (Ghosh et al. 1981) and the higher rate of this disorder among Caucasians than among Blacks in the United States (Chung and Myrianthopoulos 1975). In the case of Klippel-Feil syndrome, pilonidal sinus, and other similar relatively minor disorders the affected individuals may perhaps have what could be described as larval forms of neural tube defects. This formulation leads to certain implications. Gross failures of fusion of the two sides of the nervous system are obviously disadvantageous both for survival and for normal function. On the other hand, complete fusion does not normally occur, since most structures in the neuraxis are doubled. At one extreme excessive fusion can occur, as in holoprosencephaly, in which the forebrain halves are fused with a single ventricle. At the other extreme the two sides may fail to be connected normally, as seen in agenesis of the corpus callosum. In most individuals there is a balance between the poles of a highly unitary nervous system and one that displays varying degrees of lateral dissociation.

The possibility should be entertained that milder degrees of diminished fusion may be advantageous. One of us (NG) has suggested elsewhere that the normal nervous system is far from unitary and that a necessary condition for consciousness may be the occurrence of separated neural events with some degree of independence from each other. Mild degrees of diminished fusion might lead to the formation of superior individuals who may be closer to the goal of optimal cognitive capacity, that is, the ideal balance between separation and fusion.

It is likely that a diminished degree of unity would be present in one system but not others. The capacity of each half-brain to control its motor functions relatively independently may be one of the factors accounting for the high rate of nonrighthandedness among athletes, and in particular very successful athletes, and in fields such as architecture and the other visual arts.

Skeletal anomalies have been said to occur in elevated frequency in children of mothers who were themselves exposed to diethylstilbestrol, the masculinizing effects of which will be discussed in the next section (Janerich, Piper, and Glebatis 1974). If rats are exposed to acetazolamide or other carbonic anhydrase inhibitors, the result is a high rate of limb reduction defects (failure to form the distal portion of the limb), which usually involve the right forelimb in females (Layton and Hallesy 1965; Scott et al. 1972) (see figure 15.1). A. M. Galaburda and G. Sherman (personal observations) have found that the acetazolamide-exposed animals also frequently have anomalous cortical cytoarchitecture. W. E. Castle, in a signed footnote to an article by Larrabee (1906), mentions a strain of guinea pigs in whom the females frequently had right hindlimb polydactyly, and Di Paolo (1964) found that he could induce the same anomaly with BUDR. In humans limb reduction defects have a predilection for the right arm in male offspring. DES children also suffer from an excess of limb reduction deficits (Janerich, Piper, and Glebatis 1974). The condition of right radial aplasia and thrombocytopenia occurs primarily in males (Hall et al 1969).

Limb reduction defects caused in other ways may also be lateralized. Thalidomide given to pregnant women usually causes bilateral disorder, but unilateral defects are reported to be located more often on the left (Assemany, Neu, and Gardner 1970). By contrast, LSD produces absence of fingers particularly on the right hand.

Another pertinent condition is mitral valve prolapse (MVP), a female-preponderant condition (with a rate of about 20% in some series) in which affected individuals show a remarkable array of associated alterations in other systems (Channick et al. 1981; Devereux et

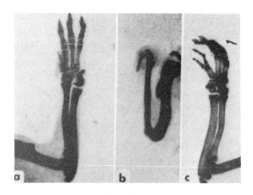

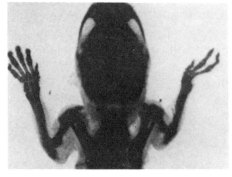

Figure 15.1
Top: Offspring of rats given a diet containing acetazolamide during pregnancy. (a) Dorsal view, right forearm and hand; one digit missing. (b) Medial view, right arm; four digits and ulna missing. (c) Dorsal view, left hand of animal shown in (b); post-axial polydactylism. Bottom: Offspring of a rat given a diet containing acetazolamide during pregnancy. Digits 4 and 5 missing from right hand. From Layton and Hallesy 1965. Copyright 1965 by the AAAS.

al. 1982; Pickering, Brody, and Barrett 1981). A skeletal anomaly (the straight back syndrome) is often present, as well as abnormal platelets and a high rate of migraine and endocrine disorders. (We should note in passing the reported high rate of platelet anomalies in attention deficit disorder (Koike et al. 1984).) MVP females have on the average smaller breasts than controls (Rosenberg et al. 1983), which suggests a masculinizing effect and therefore raises the possibility that this group will have a high rate of anomalous dominance. Conceivably, MVP is a common marker of females with anomalous dominance.

Studies of other forms of congenital heart disease also suggest a relationship to anomalous dominance. In a study of neuropsychological test performances of girls and boys with congenital heart disease (Honzik et al. 1969) the boys' scores were similar to those of male controls, that is, their performance IQ scores were higher on the average than their verbal scores. The girls' scores were unusual, however, being similar to those of males and not to those of most girls, who tend to show the opposite pattern. The pattern of higher performance IQ scores would be expected more frequently in females with anomalous dominance. The sex differences in the scores of the patients with congenital heart disease suggest hormonal effects. There is an intriguing pharmacological parallel. Sex hormone receptors have been found in the rat heart, and the digitalis glycosides contain a steroid skeleton. Digitalis can lead to gynecomastia in males, presumably because the drug or its metabolites have intrinsic activity at estradiol receptors. The possibility that sex hormones play a role in congenital heart disease is suggested by several studies (Heinonen et al. 1977; Levy, Cohen, and Fraser 1973; Lorber, Cassidy, and Engel 1979; Nora et al. 1976).

Certain skeletal features are characteristic of some forms of headache. In contrast to migraine, cluster headache is strongly male predominant. Graham et al. (1970) described the high frequency in cluster patients of a leonine facies, with orange peel skin and a full head of wiry curly hair. Kudrow (1974) has found that cluster patients are on averages three inches taller than controls.

The issue of skeletal changes has two important implications. There is a body of literature, much of it from the last century, on the association of skeletal anomalies with disordered behavior, which for several reasons did not achieve acceptance. Cesare Lombroso described an elevated rate of skeletal anomalies—for instance, asymmetrical ears—in criminals and mental defectives, and recent authors (Durfee 1974) have revived this notion. One reason for the rejection of these ideas was the observation that the same anomalies might be present in normals or highly superior individuals, which suggested that they might be uniformly distributed in the population. It is possible, however, that the distribution is bimodal, with an elevated rate of anomalies occurring both in the very talented and in the very disadvantaged, and a low rate in the general population. This is similar to what has been suggested for anomalous dominance—for example, that lefthandedness is very frequent both in mental defectives and in very talented groups.

There is also a large literature on the association of *somatotypes* (body types) with different behavioral characteristics and diseases. Kretschmer proposed that different body types were associated with different forms of mental illness, a concept that has received greater attention from continental and British than from American psychiatrists. In the United States, Draper, Dupertuis, and Caughey (1944) argued for the association of certain body types with particular diseases, but this did not arouse much attention. A typical claim was that patients with rheumatic fever were likely to have irregular teeth, but unfortunately adequate statistical documentation was rarely provided.

There has recently been a dramatic revival of somatotype studies that meet the requirements for reasonable scientific evidence. Women with a tendency to upper body obesity have a much higher rate of diabetes than those with lower body obesity, involving especially the buttocks and legs (Kissebah et al. 1982; Maugh 1982). These females, whose pattern of obesity resembles the common male pattern of broad shoulders and upper body fat, tend to have high free testosterone, raising the possibility that this group has an elevated rate of anomalous dominance. This result gains added interest from the fact that diabetes is generally a male-predominant disorder. Benign intracranial hypertension (BIH) occurs overwhelmingly in females who are obese and have a strong history of menstrual irregularities. This raises the possibility that BIH occurs in the group with upper body obesity and high free testosterone, which would account for the high rate of menstrual irregularities. If this is the case, then BIH should occur more often among women with anomalous dominance. A woman we have recently seen falls into this category, but only extensive controlled studies can confirm or refute this speculation. It also raises the possibility that the capacity of upper and lower body fat to produce estradiol differs.

Bodily asymmetries other than those of the skeleton also deserve mention. In the next section we will discuss asymmetries of the testis. Studies of fingerprints and other dermatoglyphics have shown less asymmetry on the average in lefthanders than in righthanders (Cummins and Midlo 1943). In general, lefthanders have less anatomical asymmetry in the brain (Galaburda et al. 1978), testes (Chang et al. 1960), and skin. Certain other somatic asymmetries (such as the hair whorl on the back of the head) are often said to be correlated with handedness, but they have not been adequately studied, probably because of the problems in the measurement of handedness that were discussed earlier. The same is probably true for limb asymmetries and possibly for those of the face.

Attention is often called to different patterns of folding the arms, clasping the hands, and crossing the legs; it is argued that these are related to handedness, but no good data exist. Preliminary observations suggest to us that these patterns are the result of differences in lengths of bones on the two sides.

15.3 Sexual and Reproductive Function

We have already pointed out that the high rate of twinning in the lefthanded population may well reflect some variation in hormonal endowment. Mothers of twins in Nigeria have high FSH (follicle-stimulating hormone) levels, but handedness has not been studied in this population. In Scotland mothers of twins do not have high FSH levels (Nylander 1978). It is, of course, conceivable that several different factors might favor twinning.

A corollary of our hypothesis is that lefthanded females are likely to differ endocrinologically, immunologically, or both, from righthanded females. This in turn implies that the gynecological and obstetrical histories of lefthanders may well differ from those of righthanders, and we are now investigating this possibility. Herzog et al. (1982) described a high rate of abnormal responses to luteinizing hormone-releasing hormone (LHRH) in patients with temporal lobe epilepsy, a condition in which Taylor (1974) found an elevated rate of lefthandedness. More recently, Herzog et al. (1984) have documented a high rate of temporal lobe abnormalities in polycystic ovary (PCO) syndrome. We expect an elevated rate of anomalous dominance in this group of masculinized females, although we have not yet documented this. It is interesting that those familiar with PCO syndrome report a high frequency of migraine in this condition. In temporal lobe epileptic females we have also found a high rate of benign endocrine disorders, including ovarian cysts and endometriosis. Diethylstilbestrol (DES) was shown years ago to produce masculinizing effects on female offspring (Bongiovanni, Di George, and Grumbach 1959). The reasons for this have become clear in recent years with the discovery that testosterone masculinizes the rat brain. Estradiol within certain nuclei of the hypothalamus is actually the final cause of this masculinization, but these nuclei are protected from the circulating estradiol that, in the rat, is bound to alphafetoprotein (AFP). Testosterone is not bound by AFP and thus reaches these nuclei, where it is converted to estradiol by aromatase. DES also masculinizes; although it is an estrogen, it is not bound by AFP and thus reaches the brain sites within which it acts like estradiol to masculinize. It is not surprising that DES-exposed daughters have a high rate of gynecological difficulties and infertility and an elevated rate of children with congenital anomalies, all of which may reflect this masculinizing effect. We have seen several DES daughters with features such as facial hirsutism, acne, and unusual sensitivity to the masculinizing effects of phenytoin. A high rate of anomalous dominance might be expected in this group, and our preliminary findings on 77 DES daughters support this hypothesis. In psychological studies of a small sample of DES children Hines (1982) found some results that she interpreted as consistent with a masculinizing effect on the brain, but other data summarized in her review differ; the numbers were again small, however. Further study on larger numbers is obviously warranted.

In our view it is likely that sex organ anomalies are more common in male lefthanders. The right testis and right ovary develop before the left-sided gonads. In a Chinese study the right testis was found to be usually higher and heavier, but the distribution was altered in lefthanders (Chang et al. 1960). We have heard, but have been unable to verify, that undescended testes are common in autistic children. We have seen one young autistic man with a history of an undescended testis, who also had skeletal asymmetry, a pilonidal sinus, an unusual pattern of hair color, and parents and a sibling with early gray hair. Several lefthanders have pointed out to us the occurrence of anomalies of their sperm in association with infertility. In one case the individual (a lefthanded childhood dyslexic) had a righthanded brother with celiac disease, a condition with a high rate of sperm anomalies (Farthing et al. 1982). We shall later mention Kartagener syndrome, which has a high frequency of situs inversus and abnormal sperm. DES sons are less likely to marry (Beral and Colwell 1981). Our preliminary studies also show a high rate of nonrighthandedness in nine DES males, but the sample is too small for confidence.

It is interesting to ask why male infertility might be associated with a high rate of lefthandedness (although this has not yet been documented). It seems clear that in certain conditions high testosterone levels in utero may be associated with later hypogonadism, as in Klinefelter syndrome. Furthermore, when female rats are stressed in pregnancy the male fetuses have an early testosterone surge but later have permanently low levels of free testosterone. It is possible that in certain circumstances a very high testosterone level in utero at a particular period may lead to damage to the testes in their testosterone-producing function or to the process of formation of sperm.

15.3.1 Diseases with Gonadal, Brain, and Immune Anomalies

As previously noted, several conditions involve both endocrine and immune anomalies and abnormal brain development. In dystrophia myotonica, in which there is testicular or ovarian atrophy and male pattern baldness (which suggests, in the face of testicular atrophy, high sensitivity to dihydrotestosterone), disordered neuronal migration may be found (Rosman and Kakulas 1966). Ataxia telangiectasia combines neuronal maldevelopment with gonadal dysgenesis and high AFP levels. There are several other conditions of this type.

15.3.2 Asymmetrical Aspects of Sexual Function

In several species—for instance, in most birds and in some bats— only one ovary is functional (Bulmer 1970). In some bats ovulation takes place only in the right ovary (Bleier and Ehteshami 1981), unless this is removed, in which case it takes place in the left. Humans produce ova from both ovaries, but it is not known whether ovulation is more frequent on one side or whether some women ovulate predominantly on one side. Neural control over gonadal function has been amply documented. Gerendai (1984) has shown that many lesions of the central nervous system or of peripheral nerves (such as the vagus) in the rat lead to alterations in the time of onset of puberty. Furthermore, lesions are often more effective on one side than on the other. Gerendai has also found asymmetrical neural control of the ovary. After removal of one ovary hypertrophy of the remaining one is asymmetrical, with greater hypertrophy on the right after left removal. The right hypothalamus has twice the LHRH content of the left. Whether similar effects occur in humans is not known. Nordeen and Yahr (1982) have shown that whereas implantation of estradiol in the right hypothalamus leads to masculinization of newborn female rats (as shown, for instance, by preference for other females), implantation on the left leads to defeminization (for instance, loss of the estrus cycle). Cancer of the breast and unilateral breast hypertrophy are both more common on the left (Haagensen 1971), suggesting that the breasts, like the ovaries, are under asymmetrical control.

15.3.3 Homosexuality

Several homosexuals have written to us suggesting that there is a high rate of lefthandedness in this population, but no study of this claim has yet been reported. A high rate of nonrighthandedness in this population may seem at first to be difficult to explain in the light of some animal experiments. Ward and Weisz (1980) and Dörner, Gotz, and Docke (1983) have shown that, in rats, stress in midpregnancy causes the male offspring to have permanently low free testosterone levels and homosexual behavior. Dörner has reported low free testosterone in human homosexuals, but no other group has yet confirmed this. His group has also reported a higher rate of stress in pregnancy in mothers of homosexuals than in those of controls (Dörner et al. 1983). Low free testosterone has been found in male temporal lobe epileptics in whom altered sexual behavior, including hyposexuality, is frequently seen. The low testosterone level was independent of drug therapy (Toone et al. 1983). If the situation in the human is similar to that in the rat, then one would arrive at the apparently paradoxical conclusion that a group with low free testosterone levels in adult life should have a high rate of anomalous dominance. The answer is, we believe, given by the experiment of Ward and Weisz (1980) showing that when the pregnant rat is stressed, testosterone first *rises* to higher than normal levels in male fetuses and then drops to permanently low levels. Infants with Klinefelter syndrome may also have very high testosterone in cord blood, becoming hypogonadal only later on. Handedness would, of course, be determined by the level in fetal life, and not by adult levels. Netley and Rovet (1982) have recently reported an elevated rate of lefthandedness in Klinefelter syndrome.

If the above interpretation is correct, it opens up another way of looking at AIDS. The rarity of this disorder in female prostitutes renders unlikely explanations based on promiscuity, although those who are more promiscuous are obviously more extensively exposed. One possible alternative is that AIDS is caused by a virus that has undergone a recent mutation. As a result of the mutation the virus is capable of attacking individuals with a specific immunological constitution. Some individuals have this immunological pattern as the result of a particular pattern of intrauterine hormonal experience. Other vulnerable populations, such as Haitian males and Central African females, may have the same immunological pattern for quite different reasons. Another possibility is that a preexisting virus with these special immunological properties has only recently been introduced to the susceptible Western homosexual population. In either case it might be useful to study the handedness patterns of homosexuals, and in particular of those with AIDS. We shall speak in another section about other possibilities of selective susceptibility to certain infections in the anomalous dominance population.

15.3.4 Pregnancy

Birth trauma. A high rate of difficult births has been claimed for many conditions—for example, lefthandedness (Bakan 1977), autism (Coleman 1976) and other childhood learning disorders, and schizophrenia (McNeil and Kaij 1978)—although many of these data are in dispute. The usual assumption is that a high rate of birth difficulty implies that trauma to the brain at birth is responsible for many cases of these conditions. However, the lesions that have been found in several cases of childhood dyslexia are clearly the result of alterations during intrauterine development and cannot be the result of birth trauma. It seems to us that difficult birth is much more likely to be a parallel manifestation rather than the cause of these disorders; in other words, the same influences that alter brain development also lead to disturbance of the birth process. This view implies that all, or nearly all, of the children who later turn out to be autistic would still suffer from this condition even if birth trauma were avoided, say, by Caesarian section. This hypothesis leads to a surprising conclusion. As obstetrical care improves, with a reduction in frank brain trauma at birth, the frequency of gross neurological damage should drop; but the rate of the childhood learning disorders might well rise. Children whose brain development has been disturbed in such a way as to make them dyslexic are also more likely to undergo difficult deliveries and therefore to suffer brain damage at birth. The gross impairments that result may make it impossible to diagnose typical dyslexia or autism at a later date. With better care at birth many of these children will be protected from gross brain damage and will therefore be recognized as having typical learning disorders.

Anomalous dominance in offspring. There are several reasons why parents with anomalous dominance will have a higher rate of children with anomalous dominance. In the first place, the anomalously dominant parent will transmit any genetic predispositions to factors that favor anomalous dominance. Among undoubtedly many other factors, these might include immune mechanisms and increased production of or sensitivity to hormones.

There will also be nongenetic effects. Thus, when the mother is anomalously dominant, she will often be hormonally anomalous in such a way as to favor the production of children with similar dominance patterns. The anomalous hormonal pattern of the mother may reflect her own genetic pattern, but when the responsible genes are not shared with the fetus, then the effects on the fetus will be independent to a great extent of its own genetic endowment. There will be other cases in which the mother was herself exposed to an anomalous hormonal environment, as a result of her own genetic endowment or as a result of nongenetic effects, for example, hormones controlled by maternal genes that she did not share or exogenous stimuli that altered the hormonal atmosphere, such as sex steroids, other drugs, and even the season of birth. Rats exposed to early androgens are permanently altered. DES daughters, who have high rates of difficulty in pregnancy, are probably an example of a similar phenomenon in humans. One such DES daughter, who had severe acne and small breasts, had unusually marked androgenic responses to phenytoin. The fetus carried by such a mother has a strong chance of being exposed to an anomalous environment.

Further implications of hormonal atmosphere in pregnancy. It is important to look at other implications of the hormonal ambience in pregnancy. We will consider two examples, involving Huntington's disease and dystrophia myotonica.

Huntington's disease is transmitted as a Mendelian dominant; that is, on the average half of both male and female children are affected, and the disease is passed on equally often by affected fathers and affected mothers. Unexpectedly, however, early onset cases of this disorder are overwhelmingly often transmitted by the father (Myers et al. 1983). Why do maternally transmitted cases not have an early onset? One possible explanation is that the death rate in utero is higher when the mother is affected, but since there is no overall shortage of maternally transmitted cases, this is unlikely. We will not discuss other explanations that have been advanced, but we will offer a possible alternative. Assume that the Huntington gene produces specific changes in the endocrine or other metabolic characteristics of the mother. The fetus of an affected mother is thus exposed to this anomalous chemical environment, which, we suggest, may act to repress expression of the Huntington gene at least for several years.

The implication of this mechanism is that there already exists a measure of delaying the onset of Huntington's disease; learning its exact nature might lead to preventive measures, which could be applied to paternally transmitted cases while they are still in utero. Furthermore, it is conceivable that the naturally occurring mechanism could be improved upon so as to prevent expression entirely.

The possibility that the Huntington mother is hormonally anomalous should not be surprising, since dopamine has important effects on the hypothalamus; for instance, it inhibits prolactin release. Furthermore, Bird, Chiappa, and Fink (1976) reported high levels of LHRH in the brains of Huntington females, although this finding has not been replicated.

If this speculation is correct, then the possibility also arises that maternally and paternally transmitted cases might have different rates of lefthandedness.

In dystrophia myotonica, also transmitted as a Mendelian dominant, the reverse is found: early onset cases are more likely to be maternally transmitted. Presumably the intrauterine environment provided by an affected mother permits earlier expression of the disease gene. The evidence for hormonal anomaly is clear in this disorder. Ovarian and testicular atrophy are common, and infertility is frequently present (Harper 1979). Data on anomalous dominance are not available for maternally and paternally transmitted cases.

Prematurity. From the discussion so far, the reasons for a possible elevated rate of prematurity or preterm birth in offspring of parents with anomalous dominance should be clear. The male fetus who receives genes from the father that favor anomalous dominance may be a producer of high levels of testosterone, which may lead to premature or preterm delivery. Similarly, anomalously dominant mothers may have higher rates of prematurity. The elevated rate of subsequent cognitive difficulties in prematures is usually attributed to high rates of difficult birth and postnatal complications. In some cases, however, the later cognitive problems may simply reflect a higher rate of anomalous dominance. It should be noted that prematurity is more common in male infants.

There is another reason why brains of prematures might be atypical. The planum temporale asymmetry is typically seen at about 31 weeks of gestation (Chi, Dooling, and Gilles 1977); in other words, the gyrus of Heschl is not seen on the left until that time, although it appears on the right seven to ten days earlier. Many premature infants are born before the 31st week and thus have no visible planum temporale asymmetry at birth. How does this brain develop outside the uterus? It is often said that the premature brain develops normally postnatally, and indeed even rapidly so that it "catches up" with the normal brain. We think it unlikely that maturation takes place normally, however, especially in the absence of the normal intrauterine hormonal atmosphere.

The absence of a normal hormonal atmosphere indeed appears generally to be overlooked as a possible cause of the many early postpartum difficulties in the premature infant. In the rat the final stages of development of the preoptic nucleus take place in the early postnatal period, which is analogous to the late stages of intrauterine life in the human. Since the proper hormonal atmosphere is essential for development of the preoptic nucleus, it may well be necessary for other hypothalamic centers. Its absence might play a major role in the poor control of blood pressure and other vital functions in prematures. If this were correct, it might have implications for the treatment of the premature infant.

Prematurity is more common in males and in children of DES mothers. Hyaline-membrane disease, which is more common in prematures, is strongly male predominant. Adrenal steroids play a role in this disorder, since they speed up lung maturation, but we know of no data on gonadal steroids. We have seen a masculinized female with this disorder whose mother took progesterone, which may have masculinizing effects on the fetus (Ehrhardt and Money 1967). Sudden infant death syndrome is also male predominant, and it has been suggested that its frequency follows the course of the postpartum testosterone level, which is low immediately after birth, rises to a peak in the first year, and then declines again.

The "speeding up" of brain development said to occur in prematures is probably not a true mechanism for catching up but rather a method of protecting the brain (possibly at the expense of a more refined structure) in an unfavorable atmosphere for development. DeBassio and Kemper (1982) have found neuronal migration to be accelerated in the developing olfactory system in fetuses of malnourished rat mothers. Accelerated development was found in brains of infants whose mothers were given adrenal steroids in pregnancy (Barmada and Moossy 1981). Heydemann and Huttenlocher (1982) found that in cultures of immature cortical neurons cortisone accelerated synaptogenesis.

The lack of a normal hormonal atmosphere may lead to anomalous formation of late-developing asymmetrical regions. Supplying a normal hormonal atmosphere might be disadvantageous, however, since it may place too great a metabolic load on a fetus that can no longer depend on the mother's heart and lungs to supplement its own immature systems, a problem that could be studied in the animal laboratory.

We know of no studies of brains of prematures who died several years after birth. Their pattern of asymmetries would be an intriguing subject for study. It is even conceivable that certain patterns of giftedness would be more common in this group.

One must ask similar questions about the preterm infant, in whom one might expect alterations similar to, but less marked than, those of the premature infant. Possibly even more intriguing is the *postmature* infant, exposed to hormones over a longer period and thus perhaps possessed of a different family background and a characteristic pattern of psychological endowment.

15.4 Neoplasia

Asymmetry can be associated in several ways with neoplasia (the formation and growth of tumors). Certain tumors may be more or less common in those with anomalous dominance than in those with standard dominance. Some tumors may show a predilection for one side of the body or brain.

In view of the high rate of lymphoid malignancies in autoimmune disorders, one might expect an elevated rate of such malignancies in anomalously dominant individuals and their families, but this remains to be studied. Given the relatively low rate of these malignancies, it would probably be better not to study their frequency in nonrighthanders but rather to determine the handedness distribution of a large group of patients with lymphoid malignancies. One might also raise the possibility of a lowered rate of other malignancies in the anomalous dominance population. In celiac disease (which has a high rate of nonrighthandedness) there is a higher than expected death rate from all malignancies. This is the result of an increased number of lymphomas and other unusual gut tumors; the rates of lung and breast cancer are diminished.

In Down syndrome the posterior portion of the superior temporal gyrus is often thinner than normal (Greenfield et al. 1958), and cytoarchitectonic abnormalities are also present (Ross, Galaburda, and Kemper 1984), although whether these are more frequent on one side is not known. There is a high rate of lymphoid malignancies among both these patients and their relatives. Neoplasia is also increased in patients with hemihypertrophy (Furukawa and Shinohara 1981), in whom the larger side is typically warmer and shows a higher rate of growth of fibroblasts. Tumors transplanted to rats grow more rapidly on anterior parts of the body (Auerbach and Auerbach 1982), but there are no data on growth rates on the two sides, especially in animals with known laterality patterns. The evidence from hemihypertrophy suggests that such differences might well be found.

Certain brain tumors are asymmetrical; meningiomas of the lateral ventricle and choroid plexus papillomas, for example, have a predilection for the left side. Arteriovenous malformations in the left temporal lobe have now been found by us and by other observers in four dyslexic patients. Such malformations in the primary speech areas on the left are more common in males than in females (Caron et al. 1982). Cavernomas of the temporal lobe are usually found on the left in females (Mori et al. 1980). Since hamartomas, which are embryonic rests, may give rise in some cases to gliomas, one might expect a higher frequency of gliomas in patients with neuronal migration defects. Recently a report was presented showing previous learning disability in two patients who went on to develop left temporoparietal glioblastomas (Staunton, Fedio, and Kornblith 1985). We have also been struck in the case of several patients with cerebral gliomas by a history of previous lumbar disc disease affecting the leg on the side opposite the tumor. A typical example is a male in early middle life who had a shorter leg on that side that required a special shoe in childhood. We have also seen a higher arch of hammer toes on the shorter side. All these suggest very early, possibly intrauterine, abnormality in at least some glioma patients.

Several tumors may carry sex hormone receptors, for example, cancer of the breast (more common on the right), melanomas, meningiomas, and astrocytomas (but no oligodendrogliomas) (Takei et al. 1981). Meningiomas can carry progesterone receptors (Paul et al. 1984). It would be interesting to look for lateral predilection or associations with anomalous dominance in all of these cases. Willis (1960) reported that malignant neuroblastomas sometimes mature to benign tumors, and this occurs more often in females.

15.5 Hypertension and Other Vascular Disorders

Quinan (1921) described an elevated rate of hypertension in lefthanders, but no one has replicated this study. In studies on surgical treatment of several conditions such as trigeminal neuralgia, hemifacial spasm, glossopharyngeal neuralgia, tinnitus, and vertigo by moving arteries or veins that impinge on the respective cranial nerves near the cerebello-pontine angle, a high frequency of hypertension, which was often corrected by the surgical procedure, was found in those with left-sided lesions (Jannetta and Gendell 1979). The left-sided predilection is attributed to the fact that the left vagus supplies the heart. There are no data on handedness in these patients. If the disorder on the left were somehow related to lefthandedness, this might be a reason for an elevated rate of hypertension in those with anomalous dominance; this would, however, lead to a significant difference from righthanders only if this type of lesion were a common cause of hypertension.

There is a mechanism that might lead to an elevated rate of angina and myocardial infarction in lefthanders. Individuals with thyroid hormone levels in the normal range with elevated thyroid-stimulating hormone have higher levels of thyroid autoantibodies than controls, as well as an elevated frequency of coronary disease (Masala, Amendolea, and Lopes 1981; Tieche et al. 1981). One might presume that even mild declines in thyroid hormone levels (which, however, still remain in the normal range) could lead to elevations in cholesterol, but one of the studies cited did not find this, at least not in the female subjects. If this were correct, then lefthanders who have an elevated rate of thyroid immune disease might conceivably suffer from cardiovascular disease on the basis of this mechanism. On the other hand, without considering the many risk factors for this type of disorder, one would not be justified in arguing that this type of disorder was more common among lefthanders than among righthanders.

Another conceivable mechanism of cardiovascular disorder in those with anomalous dominance is insulin-dependent diabetes mellitus, which is often regarded as an immune disorder, but we do not yet have adequate data on its frequency in lefthanders.

We have also noted the high rate of diabetes in women with upper body fat who tend to have high free testosterone levels (Kissebah et al. 1982), a group we suspect may have an elevated rate of anomalous dominance. Elevated rates of cardiovascular disorder might be expected in this group.

We have also speculated that females with mitral valve prolapse may have a high rate of anomalous dominance. This group is at risk for strokes, possibly on the basis of a high frequency of platelet anomalies.

Other types of platelet anomalies in anomalous dominance groups might contribute to a lowered rate of cardiovascular disease by interference with clotting. Patients with attention deficit disorder have been reported to have high rates of platelet anomalies (Koike et al. 1984). There is also the curious male-predominant condition of right radial aplasia and thrombocytopenia on which no data concerning dominance are yet available.

16

Other Aspects of Immunity and Infection

16.1 Localized and Lateralized Immune Effects

Certain immune disorders, in particular those involving the gastrointestinal tract and the thyroid, occur with especially high frequency in the anomalous dominance population. There might be several reasons for this. First, this population might have a high frequency of genes determining special susceptibilities of certain systems. Second, the elevated frequency of these disorders may be the result of the timing of suppression of the developing thymus by hormonal or other effects. During fetal life new antigens are produced as development progresses. We have raised the possibility that as each new antigen appears, lymphocytes are processed that recognize it as self and not as alien. Suppression of thymic processing at any given point should therefore lead to susceptibility to later immune attack on the specific systems being formed at that time. Since certain parts of the nervous system will be forming, certain specific brain syndromes might be associated with higher immune susceptibility of certain somatic organs. Suggestive data support this possibility, though it has yet to be adequately documented; for instance, migraine is perhaps especially associated with dyslexia, allergies with stuttering, and some gut disorder resembling celiac disease with autism. This possibility should be investigated in a proper, controlled study.

A third mechanism for selective immune effects is suggested by the finding that immune attack on a specific system sometimes involves a tissue factor. Thus, it has been proposed that the spontaneously hypothyroid rat not only carries specific genes favoring antithyroid immunity but also exhibits some anomaly in the thyroid itself (Talal 1977a). One possibility is that the factors that delay thymic development at a particular moment may also alter developing structures in the brain and other tissues. Another is that both brain and other tissue anomalies may reflect interference with an immune mechanism. If histocompatibility antigens are necessary for providing anchorage sites for development (Ohno 1977), altered development of brain or of other tissues might occur when some external factor suppressed the normal cell-cell interactions controlled by immune markers.

The special susceptibility of a particular structure to later immune attack, because of any of the above mechanisms, is a version of the classical concept of the *locus minoris resistentiae*, the site of diminished resistance, which has a higher susceptibility for later disease. The mechanisms we have discussed raise the possibility of several forms of the site of diminished resistance. First, a particular structure may be susceptible to later immune attack. Second, another mechanism may be operative if a particular structure is actually malformed so that it contains abnormal cells or abnormal patterns of connection, which may lead to early death because of marginal metabolic properties. Third, a structure, the development of which has simply been retarded, may contain a smaller number of cells and therefore a smaller reserve beyond what is needed for normal function. Although the smaller structure may be no more susceptible to damage than other tissues, the death of cells during normal aging will reduce its complement below the level needed for normal functioning before that of other tissues that have a larger reserve. Fourth, it is possible that all of these mechanisms could be simultaneously operative in some cases.

Finally, another well-known mechanism may favor later immune attack on a particular site. Antigens not recognized by the immune system as self need not be subject to immune damage if they are located in immunologically privileged regions, that is, regions without contact with circulating lymphocytes. The central nervous system and very likely the testes are examples of such structures. When an injury exposes these antigens to blood-borne immune factors, they may be attacked. Responses of this type are probably not rare, although in many (perhaps most) cases they do not lead to significant disease; for example, antiheart antibodies are often formed after myocardial damage but only in a few instances does a clinically significant immune carditis develop. There are instances, however, in which this mechanism causes severe damage, among them sympathetic ophthalmia and sympathetic orchitis (immune damage to the unaffected eye or testis when the corresponding structure on the other side is damaged). Certain individuals are more susceptible to such disorders, including perhaps those in whom the thymus was suppressed during the period of formation of the compartmentalized antigens.

These mechanisms have certain possible implications. They imply that later immune attack should be common at sites of congenital malformation. It is conceivable that the growth of gliomas might result from immune attack at a cell rest (it is of course also possible that the tumor grows for other reasons and that the infiltration of immune cells may be a mechanism for restraining growth). A possible example of this mechanism is afforded by a patient who developed his first temporal lobe seizure on a morning when he had an epididymitis and who was found to have a right-sided glioblastoma. He has smaller limbs on the side opposite the tumor, which favors the thesis of early development of the anlage of the glioma. Since there are common antigens in germ cells and brain (Golub 1982), it is possible that the infectious epididymitis triggered immune attack against the testis, which in turn led to attack on common antigens at the glioblastoma site. Alternatively the tumor growth might have led to an immune response to the tumor and to "sympathetic" attack on the same antigens in the epidydimis.

Other cases illustrate the possibility of attack on the brain secondary to testicular disorder. We have now seen several cases in which epididymitis, orchitis, or genital infection led to the first onset of a temporal lobe seizure. We have also observed two patients who developed multiple sclerosis after an orchitis and a vasectomy, respectively. Changes in the testis are sometimes seen in experimental allergic encephalomyelitis (EAE). Conversely, P. Paterson (personal communication) informs us that in experiments performed in collaboration with S. M. Harwin in 1959–62 it was found that immunization of rats with homogenized testis or corpus luteum produced the typical histological changes of EAE in 10% of cases.

We have also observed an apparently high rate of immune disorder in those with congenital skeletal anomalies such as Klippel-Feil syndrome, though this still requires documentation. We would suggest that such individuals will have suffered disturbances in formation in utero of other organs, which are not as readily observed as the clearcut bony anomaly.

16.1.1 Late Onset of Symptomatology in Congenital Lesions

It is a curious fact that many congenital lesions do not manifest themselves clinically until quite late in adult life. Cavernomas of the temporal lobe, found predominantly on the left side, typically become symptomatic only in middle life. For reasons that will become clear, we consider it possible that the lesions do not become clinically manifest until immune attack on the abnormal vessels causes them to dilate. The marked enlargement of local vessels as a result of local inflammatory mechanisms is well known. Mori et al. (1980) showed the remarkable response of one of these cavernomas to radiation, an effect greater than that usually seen with radiation of vascular tumors. It is conceivable that the radiation worked by means of destroying immune cells in the lesion. This unproven possibility deserves consideration because of implications for therapy. Another study (Suzuki and Komatsu 1981) reported marked reduction in the size of arteriovenous malformations and in the vascularity of meningiomas after local perfusion with estradiol. The authors believed that the estrogens favored clotting directly, but another possibility is that local immune responses were heightened so markedly as to produce a major inflammatory response with consequent clotting.

Angiomas of the spinal cord are thought to be congenital lesions, yet they manifest themselves clinically in males in middle life. A patient whose course is compatible with the type of mechanism suggested was a middle-aged man with early gray hair and a familial history of anomalous dominance. He had been suffering from arthritis coming on after an enteric infection, a condition strongly associated with HLA-B27. He was admitted because of rapidly progressing spinal signs and was found to have a large longitudinal spinal angioma. A few days later he suddenly developed a subarachnoid hemorrhage. Two aneurysms were found in very unusual locations, distally on the posterior inferior cerebellar artery. We would raise the possibility that a series of coincidences is far less likely than a single pathogenetic process that led to enlargement of the angioma and to formation of the unusual aneurysms. Cerebral aneurysms in unusual locations are well known in subacute bacterial endocarditis, in which they are presumed to be of immune origin.

Another possible example of this mechanism is the occurrence of arachnoid cysts in cases of the lumbosacral plexus syndromes sometimes seen in rheumatoid spondylitis (Marie-Strumpell disease). Removal of these cysts is not helpful (Bartleson et al. 1982). Since this syndrome is presumably the result of immune attack on the lumbrosacral plexus, it is likely that the arachnoid cysts are also immunologically produced. Both the arachnoid cysts and the affected nerve roots are close to the site of early involvement of the skeletal system. In the case of enteropathic arthritis discussed above the spinal angioma was also in the neighborhood of involved skeletal and neural structures in the spinal column and the cord or roots. In favor of this hypothesis concerning the origin of some (possibly most) arachnoid cysts is their association with many localized congenital anomalies such as scoliosis, pigmented nevi, diastematomyelia, and syringomyelia (Cilluffo et al. 1981).

Another case was that of a woman with arachnoid cysts at a level corresponding to her clinical findings that recurred after surgery (although myelography did not support the possibility that they were compressing the cord). There was a clear-cut relationship of clinical exacerbations to the menstrual cycle. The patient had scoliosis and a pigmented nevus on the left at the dermatomal level corresponding to the clinical spinal level. We raise the possibility that there was recurrent immune attack at a spinal level affected during intrauterine life and that the arachnoid cysts, like those of rheumatoid spondylitis, were a by-product of the same process.

Another possible example of the same phenomenon is the case of a patient with spinal fluid lymphocytosis who was later found to be suffering from the Dandy-Walker syndrome. It has usually been assumed that the manifestations of this syndrome are the result of mechanical effects. It is possible, however, that the precipitant of neurological manifestations is the result of local immune response. This might in turn produce local mechanical effects, so that surgical amelioration need not be surprising.

A patient of ours with a meningioma raises the possibility of a similar mechanism. A man in his seventies with childhood scoliosis and a long history of extensive vitiligo (autoimmune attack affecting pigmented cells, which are almost exclusively neural crest derivatives) had been born with a black hairy nevus over the base of his spine. He was admitted with a frontal lobe syndrome of a few months' duration as well as fluently paraphasic spontaneous speech with intact comprehension and repetition. A left frontal convexity meningioma was found that did not impinge extensively on the brain. What was striking, however, was a feature often seen with several other meningiomas, namely, considerable edema extending well into the adjacent cortex and white matter, which is in many cases the primary cause of pathological effects. In some cases variations in the extent of edema lead to relapses and remissions, which may suggest other diagnoses. Several mechanisms might account for the edema, but in our patient the long history of vitiligo makes it reasonable to consider an immune mechanism, especially since the meninges of the hemispheres are also neural crest derivatives. This raises the possibility of immune attack on two structures of similar origin: pigmented cells in the skin, and the meningioma.

Another patient with several years of personality change, increasing headache, and mild left-sided motor signs was found to have a lipoma of the corpus callosum, which was thought at first to be producing local effects by pressure. CT scan, however, showed ventricles of normal size with no displacement of structures, and, on lumbar puncture, cerebrospinal fluid (CSF) pressure was normal. This case also raises the possibility that an immune response was taking place in a region that had been improperly formed in utero. The absence of cells in the spinal fluid need not militate against this possibility, since many central nervous system lesions with significant local lymphocytic infiltration do not produce CSF pleocytosis. Another patient, with a familial history of lefthandedness, had suffered for several years from steroid responsive polymyositis. A myelogram, carried out because of new neurological signs with extensor plantar responses, revealed a large spinal angioma. This may be another example of immune attack on anomalous vessels.

If some of these ideas are correct, then the attribution of many clinical conditions to mechanical causes may be incorrect. In some other cases growth of the lesion may well lead to mechanical effects, but the change in size itself may be the result of inflammatory immune response.

Syringomyelia is another syndrome in which such a mechanism may play a role. Although the syrinx itself (a pathological cavity in the spinal cord) is generally accepted as a congenital malformation, theories of the pathogenesis have often stressed mechanical forces. Yet in some cases a symptomatic syrinx can be seen without enlargement of the cord, that is, in the absence of a dilating cyst. Progressive gliosis is thought to occur in the lesions (Greenfield et al. 1958). Lymphocytic infiltration is often observed. Finally, recent observations suggest that particular HLA antigens are associated with syringomyelia.

We will return in section 16.3 to a further discussion of why immune attack might occur at a site of congenital anomaly.

16.1.2 Lateralized Immune Responses

This line of reasoning predicts the existence of lateralized immune responses both in the brain and elsewhere, as a result of lateral differences in times of development. There are several possible reasons for lateralized immune responses. Some immune responses are facilitated at elevated temperature (Rodbard 1981). If there were differences in temperature on the two sides, as in patients with obvious hemihypertrophy, greater immune responses might be expected on the warmer side. The worsening of multiple sclerosis at high temperature is often attributed to altered axonal conduction in demyelinated regions. However, the fact that myasthenia gravis may also be precipitated or worsened in hot weather could not be explained in the same way. In both disorders elevation of temperature might favor immune attack on the susceptible structures, although other direct physiological effects might also take place.

Lateralized immune response could result from lateral differences in sympathetic innervation. Epinephrine administered locally inhibits many immune responses, and thus greater release of epinephrine on one side might suppress such responses. Furthermore, there are sympathetic noradrenergic fibers in lymph nodes that may well play an important role in local regulation of immune responses (Giron, Crutcher, and Davis 1980). It would be intriguing to know whether Raynaud's phenomenon, when worse unilaterally, has predilection for one side or the other depending on the individual's dominance pattern.

Lateralized immune responses could also occur if there were lateral differences in chemical composition, as might be expected on the basis of the postulated lateral differences in brain growth in response to hormones. In section 16.3 we will discuss possible mechanisms of such differences.

Immune disorders may manifest themselves asymmetrically. Rheumatoid arthritis tends to spare a limb previously affected by hemiplegia or poliomyelitis, an effect sometimes attributed to lesser use of the affected limb, which, we may add, tends to be cooler. The different possibilities are amenable to experimental study.

Neuralgic amyotrophy is another asymmetrical immunological disorder (Gathier and Bruyn 1970a,b). In its classic form this acute predominantly motor neuropathy followed administration of horse serum, with a time course similar to that of serum sickness, which might occur simultaneously. It is a male-predominant condition, with a predilection for the motor nerves arising from the upper brachial plexus. Because the phrenic nerve may be affected, with consequent diaphragmatic paralysis, it is fortunate that the condition is typically unilateral. Lumbosacral plexus involvement is rare, and (except for the eleventh cranial nerve, motor neurons of which lie in the upper cervical cord) there is almost never disturbance of the cranial nerves. Although this neuropathy is presumably the result of circulating immune complexes, 65% of the cases affect predominantly the right side and 12% the left side, with approximate equality in 23%. This lateral predilection is sometimes explained as attack on the arm used most often, but another possible interpretation is a difference in immune susceptibility of the two sides. It would be interesting to know the dominance pattern of patients affected by this disorder, that is, whether those with anomalous dominance are attacked especially often, or whether their pattern of side distribution differs from that of the standard dominance group.

Two other forms of neuralgic amyotrophy exist. In idiopathic cases, also male predominant, the distribution of lateralization of the neuropathy is essentially the same as in cases following injections of horse serum (Gathier and Bruyn 1970a). In the hereditary form family members suffer recurrent attacks, usually without an obvious precipitant, although females suffer more attacks during pregnancy (Taylor 1960; Jacob, Andermann, and Robb 1961). Although both sexes are affected in these families, males tend to have the same clinical picture as in the two previous forms, again with predilection for the right side. By contrast, in females the disorder is frequently atypical; right-sided predilection is less obvious, and the lumbosacral plexus may be involved.

Lateral differences in immunity might be reflected in the pattern of certain central nervous system (CNS) infections. Poliomyelitis was also thought to attack the most used arm more frequently, but the considerations raised here suggest other possibilities. It would be interesting to know whether such lateralized conditions as herpes simplex encephalitis have a predilection for one hemisphere and also the relationship between this factor and individual dominance patterns. Herpes simplex, in the form of the common cold sore, often recurs on the same side in its sufferers, and the same may be true for herpetic corneal ulcers. Herpes zoster and especially postherpetic neuralgia have a predilection for the left side (Epstein 1971). Tic douleureux is most common on the right side, and it has been suggested, although the idea is not yet generally accepted, that this may reflect herpes simplex infection of the trigeminal ganglion. Three cases, all of Irish descent, suffered from a curious condition beginning with signs on the left side, with involvement of multiple sites (Rebeiz, Kolodny, and Richardson 1968). A case of ours had the same ancestry, clinical picture, and lateralization. This may be another example of a condition resulting from lateralized infection, a lateralized immune response, or both.

Aphasia in Alzheimer's disease may be another example of lateralized immune attack at a site of congenital anomaly. Seltzer and Sherwin (1983) have found that in the presenile form aphasia is much more common than in late onset cases. They have also found in two successive series an elevated rate of lefthandedness in the presenile onset cases, with a low rate in senile onset cases. If the latter finding is correct, it will be of special importance as the first demonstration of a disorder that attacks those with standard dominance more frequently than those with anomalous dominance. We suspect that in the early onset cases with higher rates of aphasia and lefthandedness there was also delayed development in the speech regions. A patient of ours, a nonrighthander with a history of childhood learning disorder and Raynaud's phenomenon, was a member of a family in which nonrighthandedness, learning disorders, and immune disease have occurred over several generations. She manifested a progressive presenile onset disorder with aphasia as its main manifestation, along with striking abnormalities of the antinuclear antibody titer and other immunological tests.

Pick's disease (Tissot, Constantinidis, and Richard 1975) preferentially attacks the temporal and frontal lobes, often bilaterally. Unilateral temporal lobe involvement more often affects the left side, however, and unilateral frontal involvement tends to affect the right side. Mesulam (1982) has described a group of patients with the unusual clinical picture of progressive aphasia over several years, without other intellectual impairments, but the pathology is not yet known. We have seen other patients in whom there is remarkably localized progressive impairment over the years.

16.1.3 "Sympathetic" Immune Responses

This discussion raises another possibility. An immune response should occur not only in a susceptible local region but also in other locations that share common antigens with it, as in the examples given earlier. Some viruses have a predilection for well-defined neurological systems; an example of this is poliomyelitis, which attacks many interrelated parts of the motor system, including Betz cells and anterior horn cells, but which in most cases spares supranuclear, nonpyramidal motor systems such as those controlling the eye movements and almost never affects the oculomotor nuclei. This suggests that the systems affected share a chemical similarity and therefore common immune susceptibility. Amyotrophic lateral sclerosis might conceivably be the result of immune attack in much the same systems that are attacked by the poliomyelitis virus. Herpes simplex encephalitis has a predilection for connected structures of the limbic system and is much less likely to involve other regions. Rabies virus is another selective pathogen. The existence of similar antigens in chains of neurons raises the possibility that transsynaptic and transneuronal degeneration (which occurs almost invariably in the lateral geniculate nucleus after removal of an eye) may reflect "sympathetic" immune attack on structures containing similar antigens. These degenerations are often attributed to loss of the trophic influence of stimulation, an explanation perhaps difficult to sustain in the case of *retrograde* transsynaptic degeneration. Thus, in the monkey removal of occipital cortex is followed by a chain of retrograde degenerations eventually extending to the retina. Some of these effects might be immunologically mediated; in other words, following damage to one portion of the system, there might be immune attack on other parts of the system containing similar antigens.

Trauma to the brain may lead to unusual late effects that have not been explained. One possibility is that in some instances there is immune attack in the damaged region. This may not occur in most cases for the same reasons that cardiac autoantibodies do not produce unfavorable effects in most individuals after myocardial damage. Our experience suggests that this type of localized immune response following trauma may be more common in the right hemisphere, and in women with anomalous dominance, but to prove this will require extensive clinical and experimental animal studies.

The occurrence of common antigens in sperm and brain has already been mentioned. The brain and skin may also share common antigens, as is suggested by the close relationship between some developmental anomalies of the CNS and of the skin, as in Sturge-Weber syndrome. Another example is the association of an angiomatous malformation in the spinal cord and a vascular nevus of the skin at the same dermatomal level (Cobb 1915), sometimes visible only with ultraviolet light. Although these examples are well known, the possibility of other such associations has generally been neglected. The scalp has rarely been studied, possibly because of the presence of hair. There are two minor abnormalities of the skin that are usually considered to have no pathological association: the "stork bite" (a small vascular nevus) at the base of the neck and the mongolian spot (a small collection of melanin) at the base of the spine, although the latter is often found in Down syndrome. The former may reflect late closing of the upper end of the neural tube; the latter, a remnant of the neural crest, is at the site of the lower closure of the neural tube. These two locations are classical sites of certain neural tube defects such as meningoceles, spina bifida, and, in lesser degree, the pilonidal sinus.

We have already mentioned several examples of the association of various types of congenital skin lesion with CNS disorder. Even more intriguing are *acquired* localized disorders of the skin or hair in association with a CNS lesion. A woman in her eighties with a parasagittal meningioma on the right had developed over the previous fifteen years a melanotic keratotic area about 2 cm in diameter, which kept recurring after excision. A lefthanded woman in her twenties who suffered the slow onset of a left carotid occlusion had several congenital lesions on the same side: a melanin spot on the conjunctiva, a linear vascular nevus about 3 cm long in front of the ear, and a more diffuse area of pigmentation of the face. These raised the suspicion that she might have had a congenital anomaly of the carotid artery, which led to a dissection. By far the most unusual aspect of this patient, however, was the appearance of a new lesion involving the hair. During the ten days in which the aphasia was developing the patient's sister, who regularly did her hair, observed a progressive nearly total loss of hair in a circular area about 4 cm in diameter in the left parietal region. This area of alopecia areata overlay a hypodense region in the CT scan, presumably a zone of infarction or localized immune attack. Alopecia areata is well known as a manifestation of certain immune disorders such as lupus erythematosus. We believe that in this patient immune attack in the scalp probably involved a region that shared common antigens with the underlying brain.

Another lefthanded female patient developed epilepsy with an EEG focus in the left posterior temporoparietal region. Within the next few months one patch of hair growing from the parietal region of the left scalp turned silvery grey; a year later this patch contrasted strikingly with the surrounding light brown hair. A similar case was recently observed by one of our colleagues. A third patient was also a lefthanded female, a DES daughter with a history of severe acne in adolescence, thus suggesting either excess production of or sensitivity to androgens. At about the age of twenty she sustained a short left temporoparietal skull fracture, resulting in marked local scalp tenderness, which disappeared over a few months. Left temporal seizures began about five years later. Following the appearance of these attacks, tenderness returned in the same scalp region along with intermittent boggy swelling and warmth. It is possible that immune attack was simultaneously affecting an area of previous brain injury and a corresponding region within the scalp, possibly with a major effect on blood vessels.

This very small series of cases and other similar ones suggest that the hypothesis presented here warrants further investigation.

16.1.4 Tests of Immune Function

A possible objection to many of these postulated examples of localized or lateralized immune attack is that in most of these patients such tests as the ANA (antinuclear antibody) and the sedimentation rate are negative, although there are exceptions, such as the patient cited above with a slowly progressive aphasia. Although her only peripheral immune manifestation was Raynaud's phenomenon, her ANA was 1/1200 with a speckled pattern. Furthermore, CSF pleocytosis is usually absent in these cases, although again there are exceptions, such as the patient with Dandy-Walker syndrome mentioned earlier. There are case reports of migraine with CSF pleocytosis (Bartleson, Swanson, and Whisnant 1981), but the diagnosis of migraine is not always absolutely certain.

These negative findings do not, however, rule out immune disorder. In the first place, in many clearly immune disorders (such as pernicious anemia, vitiligo, Hashimoto's thyroiditis, myasthenia gravis, and diabetes) changes in the ANA or sedimentation rate are exceptional. It is usually stated that the ANA is positive in the great majority of cases of lupus erythematosus. Two series have, however, found that in lupus involving the nervous system the ANA is negative in *most* cases, unless there is active nonneural disease. Although chronic meningitis can occur, in most cases with CNS lupus the spinal fluid is free of cells. It seems likely, therefore, that when even so clear-cut an immune disorder as lupus erythematosus begins with brain involvement, little help is to be expected from existing immune tests or from the CSF. It is thus not surprising that the origin of many other immune involvements of the nervous system might readily be overlooked, even if such cases occurred in high frequency. Although we suspect that existing tests of immune function will be negative in most cases with localized or lateralized neurological immune disorder, we expect that eventually tests will be found that are abnormal in such cases. (Lupus is itself of particular interest from the point of view of selective CNS involvement. Thus, the vasculitis may well have a predilection for the posterior circulation. We have seen two cases of lupus with involvement of the posterior inferior cerebellar artery, and Trentham (1976) describes aneurysms in the same circulation. (Selective vascular involvement occurs in other conditions as well—for example, in migraine a strong predilection for the basilar circulation and in particular for the distribution of the posterior cerebral arteries. Temporal arteritis involves predominantly the branches of the external carotid artery).)

After the discussion of infection we will examine in more detail reasons why sites of congenital anomalies may be susceptible to immune attack.

16.1.5 Immune Complications

The question arises whether those with anomalous dominance have not only a higher frequency of immune disorders but also a higher rate of immune complications of drugs or diseases. Little information is available. We have already discussed neuralgic amyotrophy in response to horse serum and its curious lateralization pattern, but nothing is yet known concerning differential susceptibility according to dominance patterns.

A rare complication of phenytoin is lymphadenopathy, and in some instances the affected nodes have the appearance of Hodgkin's disease. In some cases a lupus-like syndrome is seen. We have seen striking masculinization with phenytoin in a lefthanded DES daughter, although this is not an immune complication. We have also seen both lymphadenopathy and a rash in a patient from an anomalous dominance family. These isolated instances suggest further study.

We have already noted the human CNS disorders after orchitis or epidydimitis and the induction of experimental allergic encephalomyelitis by immunization with ovary or testis (P. Paterson, personal communication). Similarly, immune attack on Purkinje cells may occur with ovarian carcinoma. We have seen a patient with the clinical picture of mild Charcot-Marie-Tooth disease who in addition developed the clinical picture of multiple sclerosis after vasectomy. This case may also illustrate immune attack on an anomalous nervous system. Dr. H. R. Tyler has suggested to us that, in his experience, high arches and other findings of possible formes frustes of Charcot-Marie-Tooth disease are common in the multiple sclerosis population. The issue of immune reactions after vasectomy still remains in dispute, however.

As is well known, slow acetylators of procaine amide are more susceptible to the development of lupus erythematosus than rapid acetylators. Studies of spontaneous lupus have apparently not revealed an elevated rate of slow acetylation. The proportion of slow acetylators varies greatly across populations, however, with generally very high rates among northern Europeans and low rates among the Japanese. We have discussed elsewhere the possibility that anomalous dominance may be high in northern Europe and low in Japan. It would be fruitful to study acetylation rates among those with anomalous dominance.

All of these questions remain speculative, but we would suggest that they deserve formal investigation.

16.2 Infections

Infections might be related to our hypothesis in several ways. On the one hand, certain infections might themselves set up a chain of immune alterations. On the other hand, patients with altered immune systems might show a complex variety of alterations in response to infection—for example, resistance to many infections but increased susceptibility to others. It would be important to follow up the possibility derived from several clinical observations that a history of poliomyelitis is more common among those with anomalous dominance. A special relationship of poliomyelitis to sex hormones is suggested by the high frequency with which it attacked pregnant women in the last great epidemics. It would be important to study not only the frequency of anomalous dominance in poliomyelitis but also the frequency of predominant involvement of one side in relation to the individual dominance pattern.

Several infectious disorders may strike unilaterally, as does herpes simplex of the cornea or lip. Such unilateral predilection might be a chance event, but we suspect that it will turn out to be related to individual patterns of cerebral lateralization. In one study herpes zoster and postherpetic neuralgia were found predominantly on the left (Epstein 1971). The differential development at different periods of structures on the two sides of the body may depend in part on immune mechanisms, especially if Ohno (1977) is correct in assuming that the histocompatibility antigens may act as markers for development. Conversely, if development of a structure on one side is delayed by influences that also act on the thymus, the structures on the two sides may have differential susceptibility to immune attack. If some immune responses are more marked on one side, one might well picture that resistance to some infections might be elevated on the same side.

Patients with anomalous dominance may well be protected from certain infections while being more susceptible to others. Those with high IgE are susceptible to allergies but may have an elevated level of protection against parasitic disorders (Marsh, Meyers, and Bias 1981), which raises the possibility that many anomalously dominant individuals are resistant to these disorders.

On the other hand, the anomalous dominance population may be highly susceptible to other disorders. We have already speculated on the possibility that AIDS may attack a particular anomalous dominance group. E. J. Quart (personal communication) found an elevated rate of a past history of dyslexia in a group with Reye syndrome. This intriguing possibility deserves further study, especially in view of the evidence that this disorder involves disturbance of mitochondrial (cytoplasmic) enzymes. We have discussed already, and will discuss again, the possible role of cytoplasmic inheritance as a determinant of laterality, as suggested by Corballis and Morgan (1978).

Certain infections can, of course, trigger immune disorders, presumably in specially susceptible individuals. It has been suggested that congenital anomalies in offspring of mothers infected with rubella in the first trimester of pregnancy are more common when the mother is specially susceptible immunologically. The high frequency of arthritis in women who develop rubella after deliberate inoculation suggests some special immunological effects. Some infections produce immune disorders in susceptible individuals; for example, enteropathic arthritis following intestinal infection with certain bacteria is more common in individuals carrying the HLA group B-27.

16.3 Mechanism of Immune Attack or Infection at Congenital Anomalies

We have suggested that immune attack at sites of congenital anomalies may account for many cases of localized and lateralized immune disorder even in late life. The modification of susceptibility to certain disorders by intrauterine events is well documented in certain cases. Medawar found that the carcinogenicity of methylcholanthrene in later life was altered by intrauterine exposure to certain antigens (Simpson 1983). Tumors may arise as a result of acquired alterations, but they may also develop in sites of arrested development, as is likely the case for many glioblastomas. Immune responses to many tumors may be a special case of immune attack on structures formed improperly during development. We have also already suggested that in certain cases (for instance, some meningiomas) the clinical signs may depend more on local immune attack than on mass effects.

Some tumors arise from embryonic precursor cells. Some precursor cells probably disappear or are sequestered early in fetal life and do not reappear in later life except when certain tumors develop, a situation in which it is useful to the organism not to recognize these precursors as self. Injection of these embryonic antigens into the fetus after immune development has begun leads to partial protection against later immune attack on tumors containing these antigens (Simpson 1983).

If embryonic rests are more likely to persist in anomalously dominant individuals because of delays in development, they may be susceptible to later immune attack in the same manner as tumors containing embryonic antigens. When the delay is predominantly unilateral, unilateral immune attack might be expected.

Because malformed tissues may also be metabolically abnormal, many may die prematurely and release substances normally sequestered from the immune system. Immunological attack in this case would be similar to that leading to sympathetic orchitis or ophthalmia after damage to one testis or eye. Furthermore, if one tissue is attacked, others sharing common antigens may also undergo immune attack.

There is still another reason for attack on a malformed tissue. We have suggested that testosterone may retard growth of certain brain structures and simultaneously suppress thymic development. Processing lymphocytes to recognize self is a major function of the fetal thymus. Since many new antigens are being formed throughout gestation, lymphocytes cannot be processed to recognize them until the antigens are actually present. Suppression of the thymus at any given point will prevent the processing of lymphocytes that would recognize the tissues concurrently being formed. Since the influences producing malformed structures are likely to suppress the thymus, antigens in these structures should be especially susceptible to later immune attack.

Many diseases of late life may thus be the result of immune attack on structures whose development was affected during pregnancy. As we have noted, this may be the case for Alzheimer's disease.

It is a simple step from these mechanisms of localized immune attack to mechanisms of lateralized attack. In the first place, structures on one side of the brain or body, such as the left temporal cortex and left-sided neural crest derivatives, may be subject to greater delays than those on the other side. Since slower development on the left increases the rate of congenital disorders on that side, an elevated rate of immune attack on the left might be expected.

Other mechanisms may favor unilateral immune attack. The peripheral immune system (the lymph nodes) may develop differently on the two sides. Other systems modulating local immune response, such as adrenergic innervation, may also be asymmetrical. Catecholamines may directly modulate local immune response or may act on the lymph nodes that receive adrenergic innervation.

Another effect may derive from differences of temperature in the limbs on the two sides. In hemihypertrophy tumors are common, especially on the larger side, which typically has a higher temperature than the smaller one. It has been shown that fibroblasts from the hypertrophic side grow more rapidly (Furukawa and Shinohara 1981). Similar conditions may occur in acquired differences in size, such as those resulting from poliomyelitis or hemiplegia. We have noted that rheumatoid arthritis tends to spare a previously paralyzed limb. We have seen a patient with atrophy of the left side, presumably from childhood poliomyelitis, who later developed many basal cell carcinomas and melanomas, nearly all located on the larger right side, the skin temperature of which was 1.5° C warmer than that of the left side.

It is, however, not entirely clear why tumor growth should be greater in the limbs with a higher temperature, which may heighten immune response (Rodbard 1981). One possibility is that this effect is counterbalanced by the tendency to more rapid growth in the warmer limb.

17

Brain Disease and
Laterality

We have already given many examples of the association of certain
disorders with anomalous dominance and of the unilateral occurrence of many conditions. In this chapter we will discuss some other
associations of brain disease and laterality.

17.1 Epilepsy

The first dyslexic brain studied by Galaburda and Kemper (1979)
came from a lefthanded male metalsmith with severe developmental
dyslexia, who also suffered from seizures. The epilepsy appeared
easy to explain, since the brain contained an area of micropolygyria in
the left superior temporal gyrus, and such malformed and misplaced
areas of cortex often lead to seizures. The possibility had to be entertained initially that we were dealing with an unusual cause of childhood dyslexia, but this can be dismissed in view of the fact that brains
of other dyslexics have demonstrated similar anomalies. In fact, seizures occur in elevated frequency in dyslexic and other language-
delayed children (Dalby 1981; Masland and Masland 1981), stutterers
(Szondi 1932), and autistic children (Stefan et al. 1981); furthermore,
in Tourette syndrome abnormal EEGs are common (Bergen, Tanner,
and Wilson 1982; Shapiro and Shapiro 1982). In childhood autism the
rate of epilepsy is particularly high. The hypothesis that disturbances
of neuronal migration and neuronal assembly are common causes of
developmental learning disorders leads to the expectation of an elevated frequency of epilepsy in these conditions, especially involving
the left hemisphere.

The fact that all individuals with learning disorders do not have
epilepsy need not be surprising. First, neuronal migration disorders
may not be the only cause of all cases of these syndromes, and only

postmortem examination of large numbers of brains manifesting all these conditions can resolve that question. Second, all potentially epileptogenic lesions do not lead to epilepsy. Veith and Schwindt (1976) found a much higher frequency of developmental brain anomalies in a group of derelicts (people with a long history of social isolation, wandering, and homelessness) than in controls, yet epilepsy was not noted in the majority. Tuberous sclerosis, a condition characterized by gross disorders of cellular migration, may never produce seizures. The same is true for other epileptogenic lesions, such as arteriovenous malformations and new growths. Some individuals may never seek medical attention for mild attacks or for unnoticed nocturnal seizures, and some may have EEG abnormalities without seizures. Herzog et al. (1984) found a high rate of polycystic ovary (PCO) syndrome in females with temporal lobe epilepsy (TLE); conversely, about 20% of PCO patients without a history of epilepsy had temporal lobe spikes. Furthermore, as we will indicate later, individuals with childhood learning disorders may develop seizures in adult life, when they would no longer be observed by those who treat learning disabled children.

It is reasonable to speculate on the kind of epilepsy that might be expected in patients with learning disorders. Since many of the lesions will lie near the left Sylvian fissure, one might expect an elevated frequency of focal seizures arising from this region. One known condition meets this requirement. In recent years there has been increasing interest in a group of conditions known under the different names of Sylvian seizures, centrotemporal seizures, and rolandic seizures. Some epileptologists regard these as identical or related conditions, although others believe they are distinct. This type of epilepsy, beginning in childhood, is probably the most common cause of minor attacks in children; some observers claim that in frequency it exceeds cases of classical petit mal. It is generally regarded as a rather benign form of epilepsy, usually readily controlled and (a particularly intriguing point) thought to disappear in the great majority of cases at puberty. It may manifest itself by sensations in the opposite face, aphasia, or contralateral convulsive movements; it can also produce major convulsions, especially at night.

The investigations of the genetics of this disorder by Bray and Wiser (1964, 1965, 1969) are revealing. Although clinical epilepsy occurred in only a small percentage of the first-degree relatives of affected individuals, EEG anomalies were found in half of the siblings and also (though less often) in parents. Bray and Wiser argued for Mendelian dominant inheritance on the basis of the presence of EEG anomalies in half the siblings. The lower prevalence of EEG abnormalities in the parents than in the siblings could reasonably be explained by the usual improvement after puberty. About 15% of the affected parents showed anterior temporal spikes, however, which led to the suggestion that classical TLE might arise late in some cases of occult Sylvian epilepsy, a finding for which it is not difficult to suggest a mechanism. A seizure focus on the convexity might eventually lead (perhaps as the result of kindling) to an anterior temporal focus in a region connected to the original location of abnormal electrical activity.

We suggest that the type of epilepsy that will most commonly be seen in the learning disorder population will be Sylvian seizures. F. H. Duffy (personal communication) has, in fact, frequently found silent Sylvian spikes in childhood dyslexics.

This hypothesis has several implications. Sylvian spikes should be more common in childhood dyslexics than in controls. Left-sided foci should be more common than right-sided foci, because of more frequent delays in the formation of the left Sylvian cortex, and the condition should be more common in boys than in girls, a finding reported in some series (Beaussart 1972). The frequent improvement at puberty suggests that even at this relatively late age hormones affect the areas of abnormal cortex that are the postulated cause of this form of epilepsy. It would be important to study the mechanisms of such possible hormonal action.

This hypothesis has another potential implication. Earlier we expressed our skepticism about the common tendency to regard minor degrees of malformation or malfunction of the nervous system as normal. A parallel situation exists in the EEG literature, in which certain deviant findings are described as normal or benign, a judgment based on the belief that they are often found in "normals." Although the abnormalities in question occur frequently in patients without gross neurological impairments or manifest epilepsy, there is rarely adequate evidence concerning learning disorders or other such impairments.

Dr. Cesare Lombroso (personal communication) states that in his experience Sylvian epilepsy is male predominant, in accord with some series in the literature. At least one series reports a higher frequency of left-sided foci, but the data are not entirely consistent from one series to another, possibly a result of differences in diagnostic criteria. Beaussart (1972) stated that a majority of the individuals he studied with Sylvian spikes had never had a seizure. In operations on some patients with anterior temporal foci Falconer and Kennedy (1961) found a visible lesion on the temporal convexity, recording from which showed epileptic activity. These lesions were often not detected preoperatively because of their small spike discharges. The surgeon could detect these lesions on the surface, but small foci of spike activity arising from deeper regions of cytoarchitectonic abnormality would not have been detected. Although careful pathological study of the excised anterior temporal lobes often revealed congenital anomalies ("alien tissue"), similar undetected lesions may have been present frequently in the posterior temporal region that lay beyond the borders of the excision. Other data concerning epilepsy and EEG changes are compatible with the hypothesis of the special susceptibility of the left hemisphere to delayed growth. In their study of maturation of the EEG in children Walter and Dovey (1947) found that theta typically disappeared last in the left temporal lobe. A study from Italy of several thousand EEG foci found that in two-thirds of the cases the abnormality was exclusively or predominantly on the left (Paolozzi and Bravaccio 1969; Paolozzi 1970).

David Taylor made a major contribution in calling attention to the laterality and gender relations of another form of focal pathology. It is intriguing that febrile convulsions in early life should, despite their generalized character, lead so frequently to a unilateral lesion, namely, mesial temporal sclerosis (MTS). Taylor and Ounsted (1971) noted the predominance of left-sided MTS in males who had their first febrile convulsion before the age of one. They argued that epilepsy was more likely to invade a less active region and that it was immaturity of the left temporal lobe in male infants that endowed it with special susceptibility. In the baboon induced seizures in early life also led to unilateral MTS, but we do not know whether the lesions show any predilection for sex or side. The findings in the baboon led initially to some skepticism about Taylor's interpretations, since it was generally believed that cerebral dominance was present only in humans. Asymmetry is, however, present in the baboon brain (Cain and Wada 1979), and probably the brains of all other primates and many other animals as well. It would be interesting to ascertain whether the laterality of MTS in the baboon can be correlated with functional behavioral characteristics in the affected animals or their families. Stokes and McIntyre (1981) have demonstrated lateralized effects in experimental animal studies of production of epilepsy by kindling, as well as evidence of dominance for spatial function.

We have found other data concordant with the hypothesis that delayed development on the left may lead to the formation of epileptogenic foci. A man in his mid-thirties with a history of childhood dyslexia suffered a first seizure that was found to arise from an arteriovenous malformation in the superior temporal gyrus, which must, therefore, have contained malformed cortex. We have already noted that arteriovenous malformations in the primary speech areas occur overwhelmingly in males and are most common in the temporal speech zone (Caron et al. 1982). Thus, in some cases the malformed cortical regions may give rise to epilepsy in adult life.

The finding of a significant number of cases of anterior temporal EEG foci in the parents of children with Sylvian epilepsy raises some important questions (Bray and Wiser 1964, 1965, 1969). The common view concerning the benign character of Sylvian seizures may be overstated, since a proportion of people with Sylvian spikes in childhood, including some without obvious epilepsy, may develop a secondary lesion in the anterior temporal lobe. Apparently benign Sylvian spikes may thus conceivably be forerunners of a large number of cases with temporal spikes in adult life, many with epilepsy. In our own clinical observations of adults with TLE we have been struck by the frequency of history of childhood learning disorders and evidence of anomalous dominance. Studies should be carried out to test the validity of these observations. If they are indeed correct, then anomalous dominance may well play an important role in the pathogenesis of TLE. We have long been interested in the elevated rate of personality change and frank behavior disorder in patients with TLE (Geschwind 1983; Waxman and Geschwind 1975). Anomalous dominance might therefore be associated with a significant number of cases of psychiatric disability on this basis.

17.2 Dementia and Other Progressive Disorders

In Pick's disease lobar atrophy typically affects the frontal and/or temporal lobes, usually bilaterally. Unilateral temporal atrophy usually involves the left side, unilateral frontal atrophy usually involves the right (Tissot, Constantinidis, and Richard 1975). As noted earlier, the typical normal pattern of asymmetry consists of a larger left posterior region and a larger right frontal region. It is intriguing that the temporal lobe lesions characteristically show a rather sharp demarcation, typically sparing an area that is often affected in many of the other syndromes that we have discussed, namely, the posterior and middle portions of the superior temporal gyrus.

The asymmetry in some cases of Pick's disease raises several questions. There are no data to indicate whether unilateral lesions have any relationship to the dominance pattern of the patient. We would speculate that the unilateral cases include an excess of anomalously dominant individuals in whom development of the affected regions has been markedly delayed. If this were true, it would suggest that intrauterine effects on dominance were not acting to slow development only in the left hemisphere but instead were acting on selected areas in the two hemispheres, namely, on left posterior regions and right anterior regions. The cases of poor social development described by Weintraub and Mesulam (1983) might then reflect impaired right frontal maturation by a mechanism similar to that causing left posterior slowing in childhood dyslexia.

There is more evidence concerning relationships to laterality in Alzheimer's than in Pick's disease. A common definition of dementia is global loss of intellectual function, but this formulation is unacceptable since different types of dementia exhibit distinct patterns of loss and preservation of function. In particular, in presenile Alzheimer's disease (predominantly female) early fluent aphasia and constructional and memory difficulties are often found, with relative or complete preservation of emotional behavior. By contrast, aphasia is almost unknown in many dementias, such as Huntington's disease, and memory is typically preserved in Pick's disease (Tissot, Constantinidis, and Richard 1975). Seltzer and Sherwin (1983) compared two groups of male patients carrying the clinical diagnosis of Alzheimer's disease. Aphasia was common in 28 presenile onset cases but infrequent in 43 patients with onset beyond age 70. Furthermore, 6 of the 28 presenile onset patients were lefthanded, as against 2 of the 43 senile onset patients. This suggests that those with anomalous dominance are more likely to develop the presenile form and to suffer impaired function of the left posterior language regions. This is compatible with the hypothesis that delay in development of the language regions on the left would render these individuals more susceptible to later immune attack. Other data also suggest a predisposition to immune disorder in patients with Alzheimer's disease, for instance, an elevated frequency of relatives with Down syndrome, who themselves have a high frequency of autoimmunity, maldevelopment of the cortex, and in particular a thin superior temporal gyrus.

Another recently described group of patients exhibit distinctly focal syndromes progressing slowly over several years; only later do signs of more extensive involvement appear. Mesulam (1982) has reported patients with slowly progressive and highly selective aphasias. The patient of Crystal et al. (1982) with a focal right hemisphere syndrome had a biopsy that showed typical Alzheimer's disease findings, but it is not known whether this type of pathology is typical of all such cases.

We suspect that these patients probably suffer from local immune attack on an area whose development was delayed in fetal life. An illustrative example was a middle-aged, lefthanded, artistically talented patient from a family in which lefthandedness, artistic talent, learning disorders, autoimmune disease, and migraine were often found. The patient suffered slow development of aphasia but striking preservation of constructional talents, in contrast to the usual situation in Alzheimer's disease. She was unusual in our experience among the patients with these highly focal syndromes, since the ANA and other immune tests were strongly positive.

Torch, Hirano, and Solomon (1977) described a case of dementia developing slowly over several years after a left hippocampal region infarction. Postmortem examination revealed a series of transsynaptic degenerations that had slowly migrated through the limbic system. This may be an example of focal damage leading to an autoimmune response to previously sequestered antigens with subsequent attack on neuronal systems of similar antigenic composition. Hamlin (1970) found that for several years after frontal lobe surgery psychological testing revealed no differences between patients and controls. Some time later, however, the lobotomized group manifested a decline in performance on certain tests. P. Yakovlev (personal communication) believed that this might be the result of transneuronal degeneration. This might represent a progressive immune response in regions connected to the removed prefrontal region and sharing common antigens with it. This hypothesis obviously requires much more study. The possibility should be considered that this type of late phenomenon may occur in individuals with a particular pattern of dominance relationships.

We have already mentioned the progressive syndrome in patients of Irish ancestry, in whom pyramidal and basal ganglia signs appear at the beginning on the left side, along with right parietal signs and conspicuous mirror movements (Rebeiz, Kolodny, and Richardson 1968).

Parkinsonism may begin unilaterally. It is not clear whether this has any relationship to dominance. It is curious that, as Duvoisin et al. (1981) have pointed out, identical twins rarely display concordance for this disorder, a situation in which the handedness patterns would be of particular interest. Juvenile parkinsonism has a distinct lateralization to one side (Hunt 1917).

17.3 Laterality in Other Neurological Disorders

In this section we will briefly list other neurological disorders associated with laterality. Many have already been mentioned, such as the left-sided predominance of meningiomas of the lateral ventricle and papillomas of the choroid plexus.

Tic douleureux begins more often on the right than the left. Jannetta (1981) has ascribed this disorder to pressure on the fifth nerve by an arterial loop. The fact that the idiopathic disorder overwhelmingly comes on past the age of fifty raises some questions. If congenitally anomalous vessels were involved, one might predict a higher proportion of cases with early onset. Normal vessels might become tortuous as the result of atherosclerosis, but this would not account for the lateral predominance. Another possibility is that dilatation takes place predominantly on one side because of lateralized immune attack. Jannetta has called attention to the elevated frequency of hypertension in cases with vascular pressure on nerves in the cerebellopontine angle, especially on the left side. He attributes the lateral predilection to involvement of the left vagus, which provides predominant innervation to the heart.

In torticollis the abnormal movements occur more frequently toward the left side than the right. Stejskal and Tomanek (1981) have shown that cases with movements to one side exhibit a predominance of induced nystagmus in the same direction. They deny any relationship to handedness, but the series was too small to permit a reliable judgment.

There is an extensive literature on the relationships of psychiatric disorder laterality. Psychosis in temporal lobe epilepsy is more common with left-sided lesions (Sherwin et al. 1982) and in particular in lefthanded females with hamartomas (Taylor 1975a,b). Much has been written about the preferential involvement of one or the other side of the brain in schizophrenia and depressive illness (Gruzellier and Flor-Henry 1979). Boklage (1984) has reported low concordance for schizophrenia in identical twins if either is lefthanded. In addition, when a lefthanded twin is affected, the illness tends to be relatively mild. Concordance is much higher when both twins are righthanded.

Several authors have studied handedness in various forms of mental illness (Lishman and McMeekan 1976). In view of the hypothesized relationship of platelet monoamine oxidase (MAO) levels to mental illness, it is intriguing that an excessively high number of males with low platelet MAO levels have been found to be lefthanded (Coursey, Buchsbaum, and Murphy 1979). Males have in general lower MAO levels than females.

Mendlewicz (1983) has called attention to a pattern of an X-linked *dominant* inheritance in some families with manic-depressive illness. An X-linked disorder, whether dominant or recessive, cannot be transmitted from fathers to sons since a son cannot receive the paternal X (although Mendlewicz mentions a few exceptional cases of father-son transmission in his series). Dyslexia and stuttering, although strongly male predominant, cannot in general be X-linked because father-son transmission is common, although an X-linked subgroup might exist. If there is relationship to dominance in the group described by Mendlewicz, it would probably be different from that of other conditions we have described.

Bakan (1973) reported an elevated rate of lefthandedness among alcoholics; similarly, Nasrallah, Keelor, and McCalley-Whitters (1983) found alcoholics to be significantly less righthanded than controls. The finding that children at high risk for alcoholism have verbal IQ deficits (Gabrielli and Mednick 1983) is concordant with these findings.

18   Pharmacology, Metabolism, and Cyclic Phenomena

18.1 Pharmacological Asymmetry

The major credit for establishing the field of investigating chemical and pharmacological asymmetries must go to Stanley Glick and his coworkers, who have produced a series of remarkable papers (Glick and Shapiro 1984). Earlier pioneering publications on asymmetrical actions of drugs in humans (Sai-Halasz, Brunecker, and Szara 1958; Gentili and Tiberi 1963; Serafetinides 1965) were unfortunately generally neglected, and the work was not followed up extensively. Other studies are cited by Newlin, Carpenter, and Golden (1981); important contributions have also been made by Gerendai (1984) and Nordeen and Yahr (1982).

The presence of chemical and pharmacological asymmetries implies that certain drug actions will vary in relation to patterns of dominance. In the studies from Glick's group rats given amphetamines circle to the side opposite the caudate nucleus containing the higher concentration of dopamine. The amphetamines must be acting bilaterally, but the net effect is to reveal only the function of the side with a higher dopamine concentration. If the dominant side is destroyed, the drug will reverse its action, so that amphetamines will produce rotation in the opposite direction.

The situation is complicated by the finding that the dopamine contents of the two sides are not independent. When the dopamine level rises in one caudate nucleus of the rat in response to blockage of dopamine receptors in the ipsilateral substantia nigra, the level in the other caudate nucleus falls. The effect on the opposite caudate nucleus can be prevented by cutting the massa intermedia, which connects the two thalami (Chesselett et al. 1983). Glick showed that after section of the cerebral commissures the average difference in dopamine content between the two sides increases. These experiments suggest that the concentrations on the two sides are reciprocally linked.

Mandell and Knapp (1979) reported asymmetry of mouse brain serotonin content. Since administration of lithium reduced the average difference between the two sides, they advanced the following hypothesis. The levels on the two sides are linked so that as the serotonin level rises on one side, it falls on the other. The system is not stable, and there is continuous seesaw oscillation. Mandell and Knapp proposed that lithium had no effect on total serotonin content and that it acted instead to diminish the amplitude of the peaks, thus leading to smaller average differences in the content on the two sides. Moreover, they proposed (as others had also suggested) that in the normal brain each hemisphere might make a different contribution to mood, one tending to produce sadness and the other elation. The spontaneous oscillations would sometimes lead to a high level on one side, with resulting elation; at other times the opposite side would control mood, thus favoring depression. In cyclic affective illness lithium might simply reduce the heights of the alternating peaks on the two sides, thus controlling both mania and depression.

Whether or not this particular hypothesis is correct, the postulated mechanism has important implications. Just as in certain cases only one movement is mechanically possible (as in turning to one side or the other), so a similar opposition may exist between different types of emotional or cognitive function. *The action of a drug might thus be identical in terms of molecular events in two locations,* yet the ultimate pharmacological effect might differ depending on the side predominantly stimulated. A substance might act on one hemisphere to produce elation, whereas the identical chemical action on the opposite side might produce depression. This principle suggests that in many cases the effects of a drug cannot be understood only in terms of its pharmacological actions; connectivity of the regions involved must also be taken into account. There are some obvious but nonetheless important examples of this principle. The appropriate neurotransmitter placed on the hypoglossal nucleus will produce contraction of one side of the tongue; yet if the proximal hypoglossal nerve were anastomosed to the distal facial nerve, the same transmitter would produce movement of the face. This principle also applies to anomalous innervation after nerve injury, but the possibility of its participation in more complex functions has not received wide consideration. It is therefore important to look at other implications.

A drug given systemically is distributed to the corresponding regions on the two sides; its net effect in those cases in which the actions on the two sides are opposed will reflect the action on one side. With spontaneous oscillations of neurotransmitter concentrations or receptors the action of the drug will vary with the phase of the cycle.

Consider the circumstance in which the drug is administered to only one hemisphere, as in the intracarotid amytal test developed by Wada. In most instances injection on the left produces aphasia, whereas injection on the right may affect the ability to sing on key (Bogen and Gordon 1971). In this case, of course, the sides are not necessarily in opposition, since singing words involves cooperation between the two sides. The unilateral injection leaves intact only one of the functions. There is also an extensive literature showing a lateral difference in the effects of intracarotid amytal on emotion (Gainotti 1972). Injections on the left typically produce a depressive reaction, whereas those on the right typically lead to unconcern.

In the normal state the drug may act predominantly on one hemisphere. Serafetinides (1965) administered LSD to patients before and after temporal lobectomy. The typical effects diminished after right, but not left, temporal lobectomy, which suggests that LSD usually affects certain structures in the right temporal lobe. This result is compatible with clinical findings, since many LSD effects are similar to phenomena occurring during right-sided temporal discharges. In normal subjects Beck (1955) found a lower amplitude of the alpha rhythm on the right and greater suppression of alpha on that side during attentional tasks. Administration of alcohol tended to abolish the lateral differences. These results are compatible with the evidence for a special role of the right hemisphere in attention and with the possibility that the impairment of attention by alcohol may reflect a preferential effect on that hemisphere.

This principle also implies that destruction of the side on which a drug usually acts may lead to a loss or reversal of certain actions. If systemic amphetamine causes a normal rat to turn to the right, it will reverse its action (cause the rat to turn to the left) after destruction of the left caudate nucleus. If the action of the drug is predominantly unilateral, as is perhaps the case for LSD, removal of the target zone on one side may abolish its effects (Serafetinides 1965). If a drug produces opposing cognitive or behavioral effects on the two sides, then the net effect will alter when the dominant side is damaged. It might be expected that if barbiturates produce depression after left carotid injection and elation after right injection, when given systemically they will produce an action reflecting the dominance of one side. Systemic effects may thus vary with individual dominance patterns. If one side is destroyed, then the effect will reflect only the actions on the other side. Pharmacological dominance might be expected when there is dramatic anatomical asymmetry at the site of action. In one of the brains studied by Galaburda et al. (1978), the left area Tpt was more than seven times as large as the analogous right area. If the two sides were similar in their *concentrations* of receptors and enzymes, then total contents of these substances would differ and systemic administration of an active drug would be expected to produce predominant effects on the left Tpt. The pharmacological actions on the right side would be revealed only with selective right-sided administration or after destruction of the left side. Recent studies suggest that the situation may be quite complex (Amaducci et al. 1981). Although the content of cholineacetyltransferase is higher on the left than on the right, affinity for substrate is lower.

Let us consider the possible implications of this principle for particular classes of agents. Because certain drugs are called antidepressants and others are described as antipsychotic, there is a common belief in a chemistry of mood or psychosis. These terms may be misnomers, however, and there may be no such special chemistry. It is possible instead that the usual actions of these drugs reflect the standard dominance pattern of the majority of the population. Those with different patterns of cerebral dominance might react in a quite different fashion.

Anomalous drug actions are well known; medications sometimes produce unusual effects or even effects opposite to those usually observed. There must be many causes for this, such as unusual metabolic pathways or alterations of biochemical actions by the presence of other agents. A drug that acts more strongly on a feedback circuit than on the target neuron may produce a reversed effect. We suspect that in many cases anomalous drug actions are linked to anomalous dominance, a possibility readily subject to experimental verification. Let us consider some possible examples.

In some cases the so-called antidepressants (for instance, tricyclics or MAO inhibitors) may actually produce or exacerbate depression. A tuberculous patient receiving isonicotinic acid hydrazide (INH), an MAO inhibitor that typically elevates mood, developed a depression that cleared only after the drug was discontinued. The fact that the effective antipsychotic agents are dopamine blockers and the finding that amphetamines typically exacerbate schizophrenia have been advanced as arguments for a dopaminergic theory of schizophrenia. Although most schizophrenics become worse after administration of amphetamines, a significant minority show improvement, sometimes dramatic in degree.

Let us now consider a hypothetical example of the role of anomalous dominance in the anomalous cases. We will make several assumptions. Activation of a right hemisphere region produces depression, and activation of the homologous left hemisphere region produces elation. The two areas have similar chemical properties. In individuals with standard dominance the left-sided area is larger. The net effect of a systemic MAO inhibitor, dictated by the larger left side, will be elation. In a signficant number of anomalously dominant individuals, however, the right-sided area is the larger one. In these people the net effect of the MAO inhibitor will be depression rather than elation. A similar argument could be applied to other paradoxical effects such as improvement of schizophrenia by amphetamines or activating effects of barbiturates. The same mechanism might account for some species differences in drug actions and for paradoxical drug responses in children. Amaducci et al. (1981) found that the cholineacetyltransferase (CAT) level is higher in the left than in the right superior temporal lobe in adult human brains. On the other hand, in fetal life the CAT level on the right exceeds that on the left and in fact has reached its adult level (Bracco et al. 1984). This means that the left side must reach its adult peak only after birth. Since a similar process is probably going on in many regions, certain drugs should exert anomalous effects until the normal adult chemical laterality pattern is attained.

Since we became interested in anomalous drug reactions, we have carefully observed patients in whom these occur, but we have not yet carried out a formal controlled study. Our impression is that anomalous drug reactions occur more often in those with personal or familial anomalous dominance or histories of learning disorders.

Those affected appear to have anomalous reactions to a wide variety of medications, and a similar pattern is often seen in relatives. Thus, a patient in whom tricyclics increased depression and benzodiazepines produced arousal had a son who developed severe prolonged dystonia in response to a single dose of a dopamine-blocking agent.

These impressions and hypotheses are amenable to experimental test. Schizophrenics who respond anomalously to amphetamines could be compared to those who react standardly in relation to handedness scores, family lefthandedness, and personal and family history of learning disorders. It would be of interest to ascertain whether there is a relationship between such patients and the schizophrenic subgroup who are said to have reversed patterns of anatomical asymmetry on CT scan. Another method would be to compare the amphetamine responses of large numbers of schizophrenics with anomalous responses on a laterality test to the responses of patients with standard laterality scores. There is another possible reason for anomalous drug responses in anomalously dominant individuals. Since exposure to certain substances during intrauterine or early postnatal life may produce permanent alterations in the metabolic pattern, individuals subjected to unusual hormonal influences in pregnancy, who will frequently develop anomalous dominance, might have a different pattern of drug reactions from those not subjected to these influences. This type of effect will be discussed further in the next section.

Anomalous drug responses may sometimes reflect individual differences in drug metabolism. Procaineamide-induced lupus is seen more frequently in those who acetylate this drug slowly than in those who acetylate it rapidly. By contrast, INH-induced jaundice occurs predominantly in rapid acetylators. Acetylator status is not, however, distributed equally throughout the world. Slow acetylators are rare among the Japanese and other Asian groups (Weber and Hein 1979), whereas in the northern European countries they are extremely common (Sonnhag, Karlsson, and Hed 1979). It would be interesting to know whether acetylator status is related to dominance patterns. The possibility of metabolic differences between those with anomalous dominance and those with standard dominance derives some support from Coursey, Buchsbaum, and Murphy's (1979) finding that an excessively high percentage of males with low platelet MAO levels are lefthanded.

18.2 Metabolism

We have noted that influences in utero and immediately after birth may permanently alter chemical reactivity. Exposure during these periods to testosterone may lead to later increased sensitivity to it and to altered metabolism of androgens and other sex hormones. Adult male and female rats normally display a different pattern of metabolism of steroid hormones in the liver. The male pattern is found in females treated with testosterone at birth; by contrast, the female pattern is found in the male castrated at birth (Denef and DeMoor 1968; Gustaffson et al. 1978). In adult life testosterone alters the metabolic pattern only transiently. Sex-linked protein, the production of which is controlled by a locus in the major histocompatibility complex of the mouse (which also controls production of a very similar protein, C4, the fourth component of complement), is normally found in the male but not the female. This pattern is reversed by castrating the male or treating the female with testosterone (Michaelson, Ferreira, and Nussenzweig 1981).

These metabolic influences may have very far-reaching consequences. We have already noted that the toxicity of many drugs is sharply different in males and females (Selye 1971). It is possible that if the dominance patterns of male and female experimental animals were known, the situation might be further clarified. Many drugs that are more toxic to males might also be more toxic to females with anomalous dominance than to females with standard dominance. Conversely, males who were hypogonadal during critical earlier periods might well show the female patterns.

Such hormone-induced alterations of metabolism might be more marked in females than in males. The number of hypogonadal males is probably relatively small, and many males subjected to excessive testosterone effect in utero may not differ sharply from other males because of ceiling effects. On the other hand, most females subjected to excessive testosterone effects in utero would differ from other females. If this hypothesis were correct, anomalous drug reactions should be more common in the female than in the male. There are no hard data, though our impression is that females have predominated among the patients we have seen with anomalous drug reactions.

Metabolic effects resulting from intrauterine influences are not confined to the brain, as is clear from the data on the female-related liver enzyme and the male-related sex-linked protein. Animals exposed at an appropriate period in fetal life to embryonic tissues or thymus have increased resistance in late life to the carcinogenic actions of methylcholanthrene (Simpson 1983). Exposure at birth to barbiturates may alter the carcinogenicity of certain agents in later life (Faris and Campbell 1981). Of particular interest is that late prenatal exposure to phenobarbital leads to a decreased concentration of testosterone in plasma and brain that persists into adult life. Reproductive function is altered (Gupta, Yaffee, and Shapiro 1982). We would expect an alteration in dominance properties in these animals. On the average, the anomalous dominance population will differ from the much larger standard dominance population in fetal exposures to many substances, and this population may therefore have a different distribution of malignancies even in very late life. We have already pointed out that celiac disease patients have a quite different pattern of cancers from the general population, with higher adjusted rates of lymphoid and unusual gut malignancies and lower adjusted rates of cancers of the breast and lung. There is no conflict between this suggestion and the finding of oncogenes in many cancer groups. The hormonal atmosphere in utero may well permanently alter expression of genes or alter genes themselves (for instance, by methylation).

18.3 Cyclic Phenomena

Another set of influences may play a role in metabolic variations, namely, cyclic phenomena. We have already alluded to cyclic variations in sex hormone levels throughout the year. The interest in cyclic phenomena, both short-term and long-term, has increased greatly in recent years, although more emphasis has been placed on the former than on the latter. Animals and plants have two major cycles, the daily (circadian) and the annual, the first corresponding to the rotation of the earth on its axis and the second to the revolution of the earth around the sun. There is also a lunar cycle, which has been highly significant in the folklore of many cultures. This cycle probably has physiological importance, but convincing data on this point are very scarce.

18.3.1 Annual Cycles

The annual cycle is particularly important in reproduction, at least in nonhuman species. Animals in the wild tend to be born in the spring.

Even though the cycles have been muted in some domestic animals, they are not totally suppressed, as is evident from the familiar association of lambs, calves, and colts with springtime. These yearly cycles may be difficult to alter. Lengthening the day artificially in stables during the winter makes it possible for mares to become pregnant earlier, but more embryos are lost. Other manipulations may be more consistently successful. When the day is artificially lengthened in the winter, Holstein cows increase their milk production and steers gain weight faster (though not when castrated, which strongly suggests that the testes play a role). It is likely that the pineal gland exerts a major control in this regard. During the dark months it is active and suppresses the gonads, but during the longer days it becomes inactive and the production of gonadal hormones therefore rises. This mechanism clearly makes it more likely that animals will be born in the spring, a useful adaptation since conditions of food and climate are far more favorable for survival. Sensitivity to long days appears to diminish over time, so that it is less marked by the end of the summer (Reiter 1980). Male rats raised in constant darkness show diminished sexual activity, but this is reversed by pinealectomy (Baum 1968), presumably because of the removal of pineal inhibition.

The yearly cycle is not merely attended by changes in the other metabolic alterations. The hyperglycemic response to epinephrine in humans is higher in the winter than in the summer (Altschule and Siegel 1951). The golden hamster shows greater thermogenesis in response to a cold stimulus in midwinter than in midsummer (Pohl 1965). Though the yearly metabolic cycle can probably not be attributed entirely to activity of the pineal, it must play a major role.

We have already noted that cyclic alteration in the production of sex hormones is likely to be important in many ways; for example, it might affect the percentage of children with anomalous dominance born at different seasons. Children conceived in March or April will spend most of their first months in utero at a time when hormones are high. Children conceived six months later, in September or October, will tend to spend their early period in utero under much lower hormonal influences. Obviously, different quarters of the year will give rise to different patterns, but adequate information regarding the outcomes is still lacking. Badian (1983) found that nonrighthandedness was twice as common among boys born in the six months beginning in September (and thus conceived from December through May) than among those born in the following six months.

Furthermore the number of nonrighthanders born in each of these months was higher than the number born in every month in the other half year. Similar effects were not found in females. It is intriguing that compared to controls, rabbits raised postnatally in darkness for seven months were found to show an increase of synaptic contact zones in the medial visual cortex and the motor cortex on the left, but not on the right (Vrensen and deGroot 1974); however, the authors are cautious in their interpretation of this.

There are other possibly relevant data. It has been confirmed repeatedly that schizophrenics are born predominantly in the first half of the year and particularly in the first quarter. They are thus conceived between approximately April 1 and October 1, that is, predominantly during the period in which the days are longer than 12 hours. It is possible that schizophrenia is more common in individuals who have spent the first six months of pregnancy under maximal hormonal influences. Mental defectives are also more likely to be born at the beginning of the year. On the other hand, many extensive studies of the birth months of eminent people have shown that they too tend to be born predominantly early in the year; even more consistently, the rate of such births is low in the midsummer months of July and August (Peterson 1979). (In all of these studies the data have been corrected for the normal yearly pattern of births.)

Other kinds of explanations may, of course, turn out to account for these data. In any case it appears at first glance that the group of people born early in the year is likely to be more variable and thus to contain an excess of both eminent and highly disadvantaged individuals. Interestingly, there is a high rate of lefthandedness among mental defectives. It is therefore conceivable that we are dealing here with an influence on the brain that when properly controlled will lead to superiority, but in excess may have deleterious effects. It is obvious that hormonal influences deserve consideration, but they are far from being the only possible candidates.

Other phenomena may be related to a cycle of hormonal changes. The rate of suicides tends to be highest in May and June and generally high from March to October (Parker and Walter 1981), a pattern that is reversed in Australia. The role of the pineal is suggested by recent studies claiming that depressives show anomalous patterns of melatonin release in response to changes in light (Claustrat et al. 1984). Data have been published on the effects of drugs given at different times of the day, but there are few data, such as the study of

Altschule and Siegel (1951), on variations over the year. Leppick (1985) has shown that side effects of phenytoin vary throughout the year. Patients started on phenytoin therapy in the winter almost never develop rashes, which, on the other hand, reach their peak in midsummer. Since phenytoin may have both androgenizing and immune effects, this cycle may have a hormonal component. On the other hand, other mechanisms may be involved. Elevated temperatures have been shown to increase immune responsiveness (Sohnle and Gambert 1982), and this might account for a higher rate of immune reactions to phenytoin in the summer.

18.3.2 Circadian Cycles

Many physical phenomena are affected by the circadian cycle: throughout the 24-hour period, researchers have found dramatic variations in drug responses, striking cyclic changes in levels of enzymes in the pineal gland (Black and Axelrod 1983), and changes in many physiological phenomena such as temperature and hormone levels. In disease circadian variations are often striking; witness the classical patterns of fever in many infectious diseases. Migraine headaches may awaken the sufferer at 5 A.M. but rarely do so at 1 or 2 A.M., the time when cluster headaches frequently strike. In many patients irritable bowel symptoms occur predominantly at night.

It is conceivable that these circadian phenomena may be different in those with anomalous dominance than in those with standard dominance. Several findings suggest laterality effects in sleep; for example, Jovanovic (1971) reports a significantly greater frequency of sleep myoclonus (the sudden jerky movement that occurs upon falling asleep) in the nondominant hand. Jovanovic also claims that a higher percentage of all sleep myoclonus occurs late in sleep in lefthanders as compared to righthanders, but this particular finding does not appear to us to be impressive. Furthermore, in the different stages of sleep the maximum amplitudes of EEG waves shift from one side to the other.

18.3.3 The Menstrual Cycle

The recurrence of menstrual periods is another obvious example of a cyclic phenomenon. Even this cycle, however, may alter in relation to the annual pattern of sunlight. Female rats kept in constant darkness do not become pregnant because the ovaries are suppressed and atrophic; those kept in continuously lighted quarters are also infertile because the ovaries are in constant estrus. We do not know of any data on variations in the length of human menstrual cycles throughout the year.

Irregular or absent menses have many known causes, although in a considerable number of instances no obvious cause can be identified. Among the known causes, for instance, female athletes and those with anorexia often fail to menstruate probably because of loss of estradiol producing body fat. In view of the frequency of benign reproductive system pathology in women with temporal lobe epilepsy, in whom we believe there is probably a higher rate of anomalous dominance than in the general population, menstrual irregularities may be more common in the nonrighthanded. We are now gathering data on this point.

The recurrence of certain neurological disorders in relation to the menstrual cycle is intriguing. Migraine, epilepsy, and symptomatic manifestions of meningiomas may all recur in close relationship to a particular point in the cycle. Although this is often attributed to fluid retention, other possibilities deserve consideration, in particular variations in immune responsiveness in response to sex hormone changes. We have now seen this type of menstrually related disorder in several patients with anomalous dominance, a finding that should not be surprising in view of the demonstrated higher rate of left-handedness among migraine sufferers and the probable higher rate among those with epilepsy. It would be well worth studying the handedness of a large group of patients with menstrually related disorders.

An important therapeutic implication is that such patients may benefit from suppression of periods. We have now seen a few such patients, in whom treatment with progesterone or similar agents has resulted in striking improvement. This also deserves further study.

19 Ultimate Origins of Asymmetry

In this final chapter we will offer some speculations concerning the ultimate origins of asymmetry—that is, concerning mechanisms that permit the development of complex asymmetrical biological structures.

In discussions of cerebral dominance and handedness it is common to find allusions to other types of asymmetry in nature. Writers refer to the asymmetrical properties of the optically active compounds first discovered by Pasteur, to the frequent asymmetries found in plants (Flanders and Swann 1977), and more recently to the Nobel Prize–winning theory of the nonconservation of parity developed by C.-N. Yang and T.-D. Lee, in which fundamental asymmetries were shown to exist even at the subatomic level. Almost invariably, however, such references are followed by the disclaimer that these physical and chemical asymmetries are not linked in any way to each other or to the existence of bodily or brain asymmetries. The fact that most natural amino acids are found in the L-form is thus regarded as the result of some chance event unrelated to the nonconservation of parity. Similarly, brain asymmetry is usually not linked to the asymmetries of biological molecules, and the asymmetries of plant growth are usually not linked to asymmetrical growth in animals.

Recent studies have suggested to us, however, that there may in fact be a continuous sequence from asymmetry in the spin of the neutrino all the way to human cerebral dominance. Although our remarks will be highly speculative, they do suggest some simple biological experiments that may supply information directly relevant to the attempt to understand the chemical events that determine the development of an asymmetrical organism from the fertilized ovum.

There are undoubtedly many mechanisms that can lead to asymmetry. We will discuss several of them, including some for which strong evidence exists.

19.1 Systems with Initial Symmetry

Functional asymmetry of an area could be the result of a greater number of neurotransmitters, greater binding, or both. It is even possible that in some cases the larger area may not be dominant, for instance, because of abnormalities of its cells or connections or because of chemical asymmetry favoring the opposite side. Furthermore, the modifiability of chemical dominance makes possible shifts of dominance from one side to the other. Numbers or affinities of receptors and enzyme activity can often be altered rapidly. Shifts of dominance to the other side may, as we have noted, occur in some cases of cyclic manic-depressive illness. Our guess is that in general dominant areas will be larger because a greater number of cells will make possible a higher processing and storage capacity.

In some cases asymmetry is present even at the earliest stages; in other cases the organism begins as a symmetrical structure in which asymmetry is then produced. In other words, the original single cell from which the organism develops may itself be asymmetrical, or it may be symmetrical and asymmetry may be induced by the action of external influences at some stage in development. The initial asymmetry of single cells will be discussed in a later section.

19.1.1 Asymmetry of the Lobster Claw

At least three types of mechanism can induce asymmetry in an originally symmetrical organism. In early life the lobster has two symmetrical small claws called pincers, one of which develops into a larger claw called a crusher, which is found equally often on the left and right sides. Recent experiments have demonstrated the mechanism of this unilateral transformation. If one pincer is permitted to crush oyster shells, it then grows into a crusher and the other side remains a pincer (Govind and Kent 1982). Thus, in the wild a chance event—the availability of something to crush—determines whether one pincer or the other is transformed. A neural mechanism is involved by which the information coming from the pincer that first crushes shells passes centrally and activates a process that suppresses the transformation potential of the opposite side. In the male fiddler crab there is hypertrophy of motor neurons and a larger number of sensory neurons on the side of the larger claw (Govind and Young 1983).

This mechanism can easily produce asymmetry in a previously symmetrical organism. It should, however, lead to an equal frequency of asymmetry on the two sides and thus cannot be the fundamental mechanism inducing asymmetry in higher forms. Nonetheless, it may well play a role as a secondary means in the process. Assume that for some reason a given area of a higher animal is larger on one side at some early stage of development. As this area forms fiber connections to other regions, both on the contralateral and on the ipsilateral sides, it may suppress some regions and facilitate others, by a mechanism possibly quite similar to that found in the lobster. As a result, a consistent pattern of asymmetries may appear in other regions. This type of mechanism would lead to a pattern of *linked* asymmetries; that is, the larger size of one area would be associated with the larger size of certain other regions on both sides. If two or more independent regions were initially large, more than one pattern of linked asymmetry might result. What kinds of suppression or facilitation might occur in this hypothetical case? The outflow from the initially larger region could conceivably even lead to death of cells in another area or to a suppression of axon formation from the neurons of that area, so that more of them disappear during the period of cell death. Conversely, the connections from the first area might accelerate the formation of axons in another area, thus giving it an advantage in the period of cell death. The asymmetry of the callosal fibers in kittens that have undergone removal of one eye (Cynader, Lepore, and Guillemot 1981) may be an expression of a mechanism of this type, although in this case loss of axonal collaterals rather than loss of neurons is involved.

A similar mechanism could be operative even without the presence of larger areas. For example, the projections from an area with greater binding of neurotransmitters or higher enzyme activity than the opposite one might favor or inhibit chemical or structural changes in regions with which it was connected.

19.1.2 Physical Forces and Asymmetry

A second mechanism by which asymmetry could be induced in symmetrical organisms is the induction of greater growth on one side by unsymmetrical external forces. This mechanism, unlike the first, can lead to population asymmetry.

All living things find themselves in an atomsphere of unsymmetrical physical forces that are the result of the earth's position in the universe and its geography. Sunlight comes from above. The magnetic field at any point on the earth's surface is asymmetrically disposed, and the force of gravity acts in a downward direction. An organism developing in flowing water will also be subjected to an asymmetrical force.

A striking example of the operation of such forces is found in the work of Rogers (1982). Since sunlight nearly always falls on eggs from above, this mechanism produces a population asymmetry in chicks. When eggs were kept in the dark, however, the chicks no longer showed the typical pattern of asymmetry of attack and copulation behavior.

Could some type of physical effect be relevant to side differences in higher animals? It has been suggested that a somewhat similar type of mechanism is operative in humans. A pattern of asymmetrical forces acts on the human brain in its passage through the birth canal. Although most infants exit in the left occiput anterior (LOA) position, three other normal (although less frequent) birth positions also occur. Some authors have argued that the position in the birth canal leads to asymmetrical forces on the brain that affect later cerebral dominance. Thus, two studies (Churchill, Igna, and Seirf 1962; Grapin and Perpère 1968) have shown a strong relationship between birth position and later handedness, with ROA infants having a much higher later frequency of lefthandedness than LOA infants.

Although we believe that the data are convincing, certain questions must be raised concerning the suggested mechanism, which would imply that dominance is determined at the time of birth. First, it could not account for the different patterns of anatomical asymmetries in lefthanders, the types of brain anomalies found in dyslexics, or the association of certain congenital anomalies such as harelip with lefthandedness, all of which must be determined before delivery. Second, it does not address a deeper question, namely, why LOA is the most common presentation. This fact suggests that the position of the head must depend either on asymmetry in the birth canal or on asymmetry in the skull. As noted earlier, the fetus has the same pattern of asymmetry as the adult; the left occipital and right frontal regions are wider than their counterparts. When the head rotates into the LOA position, the longest diameter of the head lies in the axis of the birth canal with the narrowest diameter at right angles to this axis; in other words, the head is in the position that offers the least resistance to movement. As the uterus contracts, the head will move into this position of least resistance. The fact that the forces of uterine contraction are powerful and that the head is readily molded need not negate this possibility, since even a small deviation from symmetry in the head might still lead to the effect we have postulated.

Our sugestion is, in other words, that head position at delivery is not the cause of functional asymmetry but is itself the result of the existing asymmetry of the brain, which will have a distinct association with future handedness. Since lefthanded parents will have a greater percentage of lefthanded children, one would predict that infants of lefthanded parents would present ROA more often than infants of righthanded parents. The data of Churchill, Igna, and Seirf (1962) are in keeping with this prediction. Furthermore, symmetry of the occipital lobes is found more frequently in lefthanders than in righthanders in some, although not all, series (Galaburda et al. 1978). Since symmetrical heads should rotate equally to the left or to the right, one might expect the proportions of left and right occipital presentations to differ less in lefthanders than in righthanders.

In any case there is no direct evidence at present for the role of natural physical forces in determining asymmetry in higher animals. The number of hours of sunlight during pregnancy may have an effect, but this probably acts through alterations in the chemical environment (and especially in hormone levels) rather than by direct influence on local metabolism on one side of the fetal brain. Asymmetries in plants may at least in some cases reflect the predominant direction of sunlight.

We have briefly mentioned a third possible mechanism for inducing asymmetry in an initially symmetrical structure, namely, linked asymmetry. We will discuss this mechanism at greater length in section 19.6.2.

19.2 Systems with Initial Asymmetry

We will now consider cases in which the organism is not symmetrical in its earliest stage—that is, cases in which asymmetry present even in the single cell influences the pattern of development. Corballis and Morgan (1978) postulated that the development of brain asymmetry depends on the asymmetry of the ovum itself. The concept of asymmetry at the single-cell level is likely to appear strange; even if this notion were accepted, it might still be difficult to understand how this asymmetry could be transmitted to the descendants of that cell. It is therefore necessary to specify the exact meaning of this concept.

Asymmetry in the single cell might be structural, chemical, or both. It was found early in the history of biology that the cytoplasm itself contains many internal structures (for instance, the Golgi apparatus). Methods such as electron microscopy show that the internal structure is extremely elaborate, and the picture of the cytoplasm as an amorphous fluid or gel is now completely unacceptable. Recently increasing emphasis has been placed on the cytoskeleton, the network of protein derivatives that define the form of the cell. It might be thought that the pattern of the cytoskeleton, although well defined, might reflect random events in the life of the cell, but this seems not to be the case. Solomon (1979) has shown that the characteristic shape of a cell is preserved in its descendants. An asymmetrical configuration of any cell is therefore likely to be preserved in mitosis and passed on to later generations.

The cytoskeletal architecture is determined by the arrangement of the fibrils formed by structural proteins such as actin. The synthesis of these proteins may depend on cytoplasmic genes, the expression of which in turn often depends on nuclear genes. It was once commonly believed that the cytoplasmic genes, because of their association with mitochondria, were concerned only with energy metabolism, but it has been found that they may produce structural proteins and thus play a major role in determining the initial asymmetry of the cell. The role of cytoplasmic factors in asymmetry is well documented in the case of the left or right spiraling of the shell of the snail *Limnea peregra* (Boycott et al. 1930; Freedman and Lundelius 1982). In higher animals cytoplasmic genes are derived from the mother via the ovum. The possibility that the sperm contributes cytoplasmic genes to the zygote cannot be excluded, but it is generally believed that if such a contribution exists it is very small.

It might be thought that cytoplasmic factors might therefore play a determining role in the existence of anomalous dominance; that is, dominance might be determined exclusively by these genes (Verkoren 1983). This hypothesis can be ruled out, however, since it implies a dominance pattern determined entirely by the mother, in conflict with the fact that the handedness of the father plays an important role in that of the offspring. It is also not possible to assert that the dominance pattern is determined entirely by the interaction of maternal cytoplasmic factors and nuclear genes from both parents, since nongenetic factors appear to play a major role in the laterality pattern.

It does seem likely, however, that the cytoplasmic genes (as well as the nuclear genes) may play a major role in determining susceptibilities to environmental chemical influences, and that therefore those with a certain complement of such genes are more likely to be anomalously dominant. It is even possible that all anomalously dominant individuals carry a particular cytoplasmic gene or group of such genes. A particular cytoplasmic gene complement might therefore be a necessary, but not a sufficient, condition for anomalous dominance, since many of those with the appropriate endowment of such genes might have standard dominance unless they were exposed to particular intrauterine effects. It would not be possible to account for the nongenetic effects without such a proviso. We have pointed out earlier the findings that neural tube defects appear to be transmitted primarily via the mother (Nance 1969) and that parents of children with spina bifida have a high rate of lefthandedness (Fraser 1983).

If those with anomalous dominance carried certain cytoplasmic genes more often than the standard dominance group, then certain infections that attack particular genes of this type might occur more often in one or the other population. We have already commented on the possibility that Reye syndrome, in which mitochondria disorder is prominent, occurs more often in anomalously dominant individuals.

Chemical asymmetry in the single cell might take several forms. Proteins or nucleic acids might be found on the two sides with identical chemical composition but with different conformations; for instance, the two sides might display differences in the direction of spiraling fibrils or different proportions of Z-DNA ("lefthanded DNA"). Or there might be differences in chemical composition or in the numbers of receptors on the two sides. We suspect that chemical asymmetry, with or without structural asymmetry at a more macroscopic level, is present in all cases of initial asymmetry. The lateral differences in conformation or chemical composition are responsible for differential responses to chemicals that facilitate or inhibit growth.

Larger numbers of mitochondria on one side could lead to unequal metabolic rates and differential responses to certain chemical influences. In the remaining sections we will present some of our speculations—which are, however, susceptible to experimental test—on the evolution and nature of initial asymmetry.

19.3 The Nonconservation of Parity: Implications for Asymmetrical Molecules

19.3.1 Asymmetries in Physics and Chemistry

The possibility that physical factors play an essential role in the molecular asymmetry of living systems has been raised from time to time. Neville (1976) pointed out that beta-particles from the decay of radioactive strontium, phosphorus, or potassium are circularly polarized in one direction. He in turn cited Garay (1968), who found that when racemic mixtures of certain amino acids were bombarded by such particles, the D-isomers were destroyed more quickly than the L-isomers.

For many years the concept that the laws of physics were symmetrical was considered a fundamental assumption. The existence of any phenomenon that had a particular directionality therefore implied the existence of another phenomenon of the opposite directionality.

This concept was upset by the epoch-making theory of Yang and Lee and its subsequent theoretical confirmation. In beta decay an electron is emitted, along with a newly formed particle, the neutrino, which spins at right angles to the direction of movement. Standard assumptions of symmetry led physicists to expect that equal numbers of neutrinos with left- and right-sided spins would be produced. It was found, however, that the neutrinos are all "lefthanded": as they move toward the observer, they all spin clockwise, while the emitted electrons spin the opposite way. The asymmetrical spins of the particles emitted in beta decay might at first appear to be of little consequence outside the physics of elementary particles. It has been argued on theoretical grounds, however, that the bombardment of a mixture of equal amounts of L- and D-amino acids by such asymmetrical electrons would lead to differential ionization and therefore to greater prevalence of the L-forms. Preliminary experimental data appear to support this conclusion (Garay 1968).

19.3.2 Structural Proteins

Neville (1976) called attention to the fact that alpha-helixes formed by L-amino acids have a righthanded twist; superhelixes formed from such proteins have the opposite chirality. He also pointed out that if all the helical components in what appeared at first to be a symmetrical biological structure consisted of sterically similar compounds, then despite apparent macroscopic symmetry one would find asymmetry at the molecular level. Compounds on opposite sides of the structure would twist in the same direction and would not necessarily be mirror images. This is easily visualized by considering spiraling molecules on the two sides, which are oriented vertically. Neville went on to point out that if the taste receptors on the two sides of the tongue were mirror images, then sucrose, a steric compound, could bind to only one side and would thus taste sweet on only one side.

Helicity or direction of twist is probably critical, since certain structural fibrous compounds grow in the form of a coil. As the coil moves forward, the tip may move clockwise or counterclockwise. Such structural proteins play a role in many structures; the growing neurite contains actin, for instance, and the mitotic spindle appears to contain dynein. The flagella of the sperm, which determine its movement, also show a definite directionality, and the bronchial cilia beat in the same direction and thus help to clear small particles. Neville pointed out that in order to avoid entanglement, the flagella of a bacterium must have the same twist and the same direction of rotation. It appears likely that cilia must contain structural proteins, the fibrils of which have a consistent torque. When such a coordinated pattern is absent, as in Kartagener syndrome, a high rate of respiratory infections is found, as well as an elevated rate of infertility resulting from abnormality of the flagella in the sperm. Patients with this syndrome also manifest dextrocardia or situs inversus. This raises the possibility that if the spiraling of structural proteins is abnormal, laterality may also be disturbed. The same situation exists in the growth of the nervous system. Heacock and Agranoff (1977) have found that the neurites from goldfish retinal neurons in culture grow consistently in a clockwise direction, regardless of whether they come from the right or the left eye, suggesting that all the structural proteins have been coded to twist in the same direction.

19.4 Asymmetrical Chemical Effects

The structural properties of proteins are ultimately determined by the helix of DNA. Recently a new form has been discovered, namely, Z-DNA, which has a lefthanded helix (Rich 1982) rather than the right-handed helix that had been thought for many years to be the only form. Z-DNA has now been found in many locations, and research on its functions is proceeding actively. It should be stressed that although it has a lefthanded helix, it is not a mirror image of the standard molecule. It is therefore unlikely that it codes for proteins of conformations opposite to those of the standard forms.

We have postulated that certain hormones exert different effects on the two sides of the developing nervous system and the neural crest. How, in fact, could a compound affect growth differentially on opposite sides? The simplest mechanism would involve chemical differences in the corresponding structures. The sex hormones themselves are stereoisomeric compounds. Estradiol-17-beta has much greater estrogenic effect than the alpha isomer, which differs in the steric conformation of one hydroxyl group; the 17-beta form of testosterone is similarly more active than the 17-alpha form. Conceivably, testosterone might have much greater chemical affinity for a compound with a torque in one direction than for one with a torque in the opposite direction. This situation might arise if on one side of the brain there were neurites with one orientation and on the other side neurites with the opposite orientation, each with a differential sensitivity to sex hormones. The action of testosterone might be indirect; for example, it might act on a steric compound, which in turn would act on the actin helix. It is known that Z-DNA differs from the corresponding standard form in its chemical reactivity, since antibodies can be made specifically against it. Differences in chemical structure on the two sides could thus ensure that certain compounds had differential lateral effects on growth. Such a mechanism would be particularly necessary in the brain, in which the growth of paired structures must be modified differentially for the development of cerebral dominance. Similar situations may exist elsewhere in other paired organs.

Another possibility is that those forms of certain stereoisomeric compounds that are usually regarded as inactive might in fact have important asymmetrical growth effects in development. The 17-alpha form of estradiol is not found in the human but is found in other species; it is said to have measurable activity in certain test systems for estrogenic action. By contrast, 17-alpha-testosterone (epitestosterone) is found in appreciable quantities in humans, but no function has ever been established for it. Is it possible that, although it may have little effect on peripheral androgen-sensitive systems, it is important in the mechanisms of asymmetry in development? Conceivably, it might have a greater affinity for compounds in a particular conformation than for those in the more common 17-beta form. Testosterone has important effects on skeletal muscle, which contains a high concentration of actin, as well as on neurites (Toran-Allerand 1978), which also contain actin. Is it conceivable that the two forms of testosterone might have differential effects on actin in the neurites of the developing brain on the two sides, if the proportion of fibrils spiraling in opposite directions was different on the two sides? This is highly speculative but amenable to some simple experimental tests.

Mechanisms of the type we have discussed might fail in certain ways. Afzelius and Eliasson (1979) have pointed out that the pattern of the fibrils in cilia may play a major role in determining laterality. They also stress the role of such fibrils in the mitotic spindle. As mentioned earlier, in Kartagener syndrome there is some mechanism that leads to formation of fibrils with anomalous helical patterns. Consequently, the orientation of the cilia in the bronchi may be random, and there may be a high rate of anomalies of the celia of the sperm; moreover, as a result of their disordered pattern or orientation, it is possible that these fibrils fail to guide development of bodily organs in the correct lateral orientation. If alterations in the spiraling of fibrils played a role in determining laterality, then one might expect to find evidence of anomalous formation of the fibrils of proteins involved in structure and motility in elevated frequency in the anomalous dominance population. We pointed out earlier the high rate of abnormal sperm in patients with celiac disease. A lefthanded adult who had been a childhood dyslexic had abnormal sperm—and a righthanded brother with celiac disease (P. Behan and N. Geschwind, personal observations). We have also commented on the possibility of a high rate of infertility in the anomalous dominance population.

The previously discussed locus T of the major histocompatibility complex is a set of genes that might be related to proteins involved in motility. A sperm that carries the allele t is much more likely to impregnate the ovum than one that does not. This accounts for the fact that *t* is transmitted to much more than half the offspring of a *t*-bearing father. It has been suggested that this is because the sperm bearing *t* swims more rapidly. If this were the case, it would suggest that *t* might play some important role in the formation of the structural proteins of the cilia.

19.5 Asymmetry in Unicellular Organisms

We have noted that we support the view of Corballis and Morgan (1978) that asymmetry may be coded in the organism at its most elementary stage. This asymmetry might be coded in the cytoskeleton of the single cell, a process in which cytoplasmic genes perhaps play a role.

Although the concept of asymmetry of *function* in a single cell might at first seem difficult to accept, the existence of such asymmetry appears to be well documented. In a remarkable paper Schaeffer (1928) pointed out the striking asymmetries of unicellular organisms. He cited data on 162 species of ciliates, which in swimming rotate around the long axis of the body; each species of ciliate rotates in only one direction. Jennings had found that 100 species rotated to the right and that 62 rotated to the left. Schaeffer found over many hours of observation that amoebas swim around a glass rod more frequently in one direction than the other. He gave many other examples of such preferred rotational directions in unicellular organisms and in multicellular invertebrate species such as the Polo worm in which all members rotate on the long axis in the same orientation. He also discussed asymmetry of rotation in sperm, but gave no details.

These patterns imply that the proteins underlying motility probably have a preferential helix in each of the species involved. There is thus no a priori reason to reject the possibility that similar structures are present in the ovum, the sperm, and the zygote. We would also suggest that asymmetries in the plant world may have similar fundamental mechanisms and that therefore studies in plants may give valuable insights into the mechanisms of asymmetry even in humans. Far from being confined to humans, asymmetries of structure and function are widespread, possibly even universal, properties of living things in both the plant and the animal kingdoms. They are present in unicellular organisms as well as in the most complex multicellular forms.

19.6 Secondary Mechanisms of Asymmetry

19.6.1 Shifts of Dominance

Several mechanisms can play a role in determining the final pattern of asymmetry in an initially asymmetrical organism. We have presented evidence that asymmetry favoring certain brain regions is present early in fetal life. Since we believe that initial asymmetry implies the presence of chemical asymmetry, it is possible to alter the fundamental pattern. Because chemical difference almost always implies immunological difference, it might lead to slowing of growth on one side. Hormones or other substances might act directly on nerve cells or neurites or might modify immune effects.

Our hypothesis, based on the currently available evidence, is that the brain has intrinsic strong left hemisphere language and motor dominance and that influences in utero can slow development of the structures underlying these functions on the left side, thus diminishing the magnitude of these lateralizations. Slowing on the left indirectly leads to diminished cell death on the right and therefore eventually to increased size of areas on that side. With exaggerated slowing the two sides tend to become more symmetrical; in such cases dominance will be random. A less common effect is a shift to the point where the structures on the right are actually larger than those on the left.

There is another possible mechanism for random dominance. In animals with situs inversus (Layton 1976) the genetic abnormality appears to lead not to reverse situs but to random situs, so that only half of the bearers of the genetic pattern actually show reverse situs. The same mechanism is probably operative in humans. In Kartagener syndrome dextrocardia or reverse situs occurs in many cases but is lacking in many others. This again suggests that situs is random in this situation. Afzelius and Eliasson (1979) have argued that the mechanism that leads to ciliary abnormality in the bronchi and sperm also leads to the anomaly of lateralization of the internal organs. We suspect that anomalous dominance will be present in elevated frequency in this population.

Annett was the first to suggest that most lefthandedness is the result of a mechanism in which brain laterality is randomly determined. According to her theory, some individuals carry a right-shift gene that increases the probability of left hemisphere dominance for language and speech. In the absence of this gene laterality for these functions is randomly determined.

As we have stressed before, our hypothesis differs from Annett's in one respect. We have accepted what we consider to be the major and seminal contribution of her theory, that there is a group of individuals with random dominance. We believe, however, that the system in its initial stages possesses asymmetry favoring the language and motor regions of the left hemisphere and that influences that allay development of these regions on the left can drive the system to symmetry. Whereas Annett argues for right-shift influences, which can drive the system from randomness to left dominance, we argue for left-shift influences (as proposed by Corballis and Morgan), which drive the system to symmetry. Reverse asymmetry is uncommon. An important reason for our formation is the fact that fetal brains at very early stages typically show asymmetry favoring the left side.

It is possible, however, that there is a greater variety of initial states than we have assumed. Though it seems clear that most brains display initial asymmetry favoring the left side, the possibility must be considered that in some cases the initial state is one of symmetry or even reverse asymmetry. Obviously, it would be important to determine how often these initial states occur. This could be done straightforwardly by examining large numbers of brains of fetuses, at, let us say, at most five months gestational age, and determining how many show the typical pattern of asymmetry in the Sylvian fissures and more marked development of cortical markings on the right. If individuals with reverse cerebral asymmetry existed, they would exhibit reversal of the usual Sylvian asymmetry and more rapid cortical development on the left. Those without asymmetry would have Sylvian fissures of equal height and equally rapid development of cortical markings on the two sides. We would predict that the number of such cases would be small, but the study is an important one to undertake.

If brains with initial symmetry or reverse asymmetry existed, it would be important to know what effect the delaying influences would have. It is conceivable that in the cases of initial reverse asymmetry environmental influences in utero would lead to slowing on the right rather than on the left. A certain percentage of these cases would therefore be shifted to symmetry and some even to left-sided dominance. Conceivably, brains with initial symmetry might lack chemical asymmetry and might therefore remain symmetrical. If the pattern of hormonal influences were the same as those in the cases with normal brain asymmetry, then males with initial reverse asymmetry would more often be shifted to symmetry or reversal. If this were true, then we would expect more females among those with strong asymmetries favoring the left hemisphere, as is suggested by the higher average levels of verbal skills among females and their higher rate of strong righthandedness, and also more females in the small group with strong asymmetries favoring the right side. Wada, Clarke, and Hamm (1975) found that a larger right planum temporale was more common in females than males.

The questions raised in this section are important ones that can be answered only by examining large numbers of early fetal brains. We would like to stress, however, that even if a subgroup of brains was found with initial symmetry or reverse asymmetry, we would not accept a claim that the eventual pattern of laterality is fully determined by the initial pattern of symmetry or asymmetry. Our basic hypothesis is that there is an initial pattern that is capable of undergoing major modifications by environmental influences. It would remain the same even if several different initial patterns were found to exist. Without involving environmental effects, it would not be possible to explain either the larger numbers of males with anomalous dominance and learning disorders or the elevated rate of anomalous dominance among both monozygotic and dizygotic twins.

19.6.2 Linked Asymmetries

A *linked asymmetry* is neither present initially nor induced in an initially symmetrical structure by physical forces. Instead, it is induced in a given structure as the result of the appearance or modification of asymmetry in another structure.

We have already discussed two mechanisms of linked asymmetry. When development of certain structures in the left hemisphere is slowed, the opposite homologous areas become larger—the result, we have suggested, of diminished cell death.

As a result of the changes that occur in the nervous system when one pincer of a lobster enlarges, the neural system controlling the other pincer is in some way inhibited, thus preventing it from undergoing a similar transformation. We have already discussed the possibility that similar mechanisms could conceivably produce patterns of linked asymmetries in higher animals as well.

We have suggested that the slowing of growth of one particular region leads not only to enlargement of the opposite homologous area but also to enlargement of adjacent uninvolved regions, as shown by the work of Goldman (1978). It seems likely that the effects of change in one region may be seen not only in immediately adjacent structures but also in structures at a distance from the site of slowing or damage, a possibility also suggested by the work of Goldman.

The existence of linked asymmetries raises the question of whether there is only one primary asymmetry in the human brain, all the others being secondary linked asymmetries, or whether there are several primary asymmetries, each of which may induce linked asymmetries.

The absence of linkage between two asymmetries is suggested when one may be altered independently of the other. Thus, although the great majority of humans have a particular configuration of the thoracic and abdominal organs, dextrocardia is occasionally found in the absence of reversal of the abdominal organs. On the other hand, it is extremely rare to find, let us say, an isolated shift of the spleen. This suggests that asymmetries of the abdominal organs are linked, but that cardiac asymmetry is independent.

It is important to be aware, however, that if two functions are controlled by opposite hemispheres, this need not rule out linkage of the underlying anatomical or chemical asymmetry. When corresponding areas are anatomically symmetrical, the mechanism suggested by Annett is operative; that is, dominance for the function subserved by the areas is probably random. Hence, when two homologous areas on opposite sides are symmetrical, the areas linked to this pair will also be symmetrical. The functions subserved by the different areas will, however, be randomly controlled by either hemisphere. The final decision on the existence of linkage may therefore require understanding the anatomical or chemical asymmetries in addition to the functional asymmetry.

Sufficient data are therefore not yet available to determine whether any brain asymmetries are linked. Language and motor dominance may be located in opposite hemispheres, but linkage cannot be excluded with certainty for the reasons just given. On the other hand, it is clear that the typical dominance functions of the right hemisphere rarely shift, even when language is shifted, suggesting that at least one of the right brain asymmetries is not linked to language.

Some anatomical data concerning linkage are available. In a study of East African skulls frontal, occipital, and parietal petalias were combined randomly, suggesting an absence of linkage (Gundara and Zivanovic 1968). It would be important to carry out an extensive study with radiological methods. By contrast, Glick, Ross, and Hough (1982) found that in the human brain several chemical asymmetries are indeed linked, and Eidelberg and Galaburda (1984) found that language-related areas have linked asymmetries.

It is likely that partially linked asymmetries are often present. In this case the initial asymmetries of two areas may be determined independently, yet a change in one of these areas may secondarily influence the development of others.

19.6.3 Postnatal Effects

We have discussed elsewhere possible postnatal influences in the modification of asymmetry. Much less is known about these, although many of the considerations that apply to prenatal influences probably apply to postnatal influences as well.

19.7 Conclusion

The speculations in these pages are presented not through the conviction that they necessarily represent the true origins of asymmetry but rather because the realization that cerebral dominance is a biological problem makes it necessary to consider its ultimate cellular origins. The application of the techniques of molecular biology and genetics to this as yet unexplored area will surely lead to dramatic findings and to far more sophisticated theories based on solid experimental data. We hope that our speculations will help to stimulate research. We have stressed the existence of asymmetries even at the single-cell level, because significant information may come from even the lowliest forms of animal life and from plants. It has become evident in recent years that biological mechanisms of importance in higher animals often embody processes found in very primitive forms. Until very recently dominance was thought to be a feature only of humans, but it is now known that this is not the case. Understanding the ultimate origins of asymmetry will require studying not only the foundations of biology but very possibly also those of physics itself.

References

Aase, J. N., and D. W. Smith (1970). Facial asymmetry and abnormalities of palms and ears: A dominantly inherited developmental syndrome. *J Ped* 76:928–930.

Afzelius, B. A., P. Camner, R. Eliasson, et al. (1978). Kartagener's syndrome does exist. *Lancet* 2:950.

Afzelius, B. A., and R. Eliasson (1979). Flagellar mutants in man: On the heterogeneity of the immotile-cilia syndrome. *J Ultrastructure Res* 69:43–52.

Alderman, A. L. (1935). The determination of the eye in the anuran Hyla regilla. *J Exp Zool* 70:205–232.

Alexander, M. A., W. H. Bunch, and S. O. Ebbesson (1972). Can experimental dorsal rhizotomy produce scoliosis? *J Bone Joint Surg* 54A:1509–1513.

Altschule, M. D., and E. P. Siegel (1951). Inadequacy of the glycemic reaction to epinephrine as a measure of hepatic glycogen. *Am J Med Sci* 222:50–53.

Amaducci, L., S. Sorbi, A. Albanese, et al. (1981). Choline acetyltransferase (ChAT) activity differs in right and left human temporal lobes. *Neurology* 31:799–805.

Andrews, P. W., and P. M. Goodfellow (1982). Analysing the mouse T/E complex. *Nature* 299:296–297.

Annett, M. (1970). A classification of hand preference by association analysis. *Br J Psychol* 61:303–321.

Annett, M. (1978a). Genetic and non-genetic differences on handedness. *Behav Genet* 8:227–249.

Annett, M. (1978b). *A single gene explanation of right and lefthandedness and brainedness.* Lancaster Polytechnic, Coventry.

Annett, M., and D. Kilshaw (1982). Mathematical ability and lateral asymmetry. *Cortex* 18:547–568.

Assemany, S. R., R. L. Neu, and L. I. Gardner (1970). Deformities in a child whose mother took L.S.D. *Lancet* 1:1290.

Auerbach, R., and W. Auerbach (1982). Regional differences in the growth of normal and neoplastic cells. *Science* 215:127–134.

Badian, N. A. (1983). Birth order, maternal age, season of birth, and handedness. *Cortex* 19:451–463.

Bakan, P. (1971). Handedness and birth order. *Nature* 229:195.

Bakan, P. (1973). Lefthandedness and alcoholism. *Percept Mot Skills* 36:514.

Bakan, P. (1977). Left-handedness and birth order revisited. *Neuropsychologia* 15:837–839.

Bakwin, H. (1973). Reading disability in twins. *Develop Med Child Neurol* 15:184–187.

Balthasar, K. (1957). Über das anatomische Substrat der generalisierten Tic-Krankheit (maladie des tics, Gilles de la Tourette): Entwicklungshemmung des corpus striatum. *Archiv Psychiat, Berl* 195:531–549.

Barbas, G., W. S. Matthews, and M. Ferrari (1983). Minor diagnostic criteria in childhood migraine. *Ann Neurol* 14:364.

Bardin, C. W., and J. F. Catterall (1981). Testosterone: A major determinant of extragenital sexual dimorphism. *Science* 211:1285–1294.

Barmada, M. A., and J. Moossy (1981). Advanced cerebral maturation with intrauterine growth retardation. *Neurology* 31:163.

Bartleson, J. D., M. D. Cohen, T. M. Harrington, et al. (1982). Cauda equina syndrome secondary to longstanding ankylosing spondylitis. *Ann Neurol* 12:77.

Bartleson, J. D., J. W. Swanson, and J. P. Whisnant (1981). A migrainous syndrome with cerebrospinal fluid pleocytosis. *Neurology* 31:125–162.

Baum, M. J. (1968). Pineal gland: Influence on development of copulation in male rats. *Science* 162:586–587.

Beaussart, M. (1972). Benign epilepsy of children with Rolandic (centro-temporal) paroxysmal foci. *Epilepsia* 13:795–811.

Beck, E. (1955). Typologie des Gehirns am Beispiel des dorsalen menschlichen Schläfenappens nebst weiteren Beiträge zur Frage der Links–Rechtshirnigkeit. *Dtsch Z Nervenheilk* 173:267–308.

Beer, A. E., and R. E. Billingham (1976). *The Immunobiology of Mammalian Reproduction.* Englewood Cliffs, N.J.: Prentice-Hall.

Benbow, C. P., and J. C. Stanley (1980). Sex differences in mathematical ability: Fact or artifact? *Science* 210:1262–1264.

Benbow, C. P., and J. C. Stanley (1983). Sex differences in mathematical reasoning ability: More facts. *Science* 222:1029–1031.

Benson, D. F., and N. Geschwind (1969). The alexias. In *Handbook of Clinical Neurology.* Vol. 4: *Disorders of Speech, Perception, and Symbolic Behavior,* P. J. Vinken and G. W. Bruyn, eds., 112–140. Amsterdam: North-Holland.

Benson, D. F., and N. Geschwind (1970). Developmental Gerstmann syndrome. *Neurology* 20:293–298.

Benton, A. L. (1979). Visuoperceptive, visuospatial, and visuoconstructive disorders. In *Clinical Neuropsychology*, K. Heilman and E. Valenstein, eds., 186–223. New York: Oxford University Press.

Benton, A. L., R. Meyers, and G. J. Polder (1962). Some aspects of handedness. *Psychiatr Neurol (Basal)* 144:321–337.

Beral, V., and L. Colwell (1981). Randomised trial of high doses of stilboestrol and ethisterone therapy in pregnancy: Long-term follow-up of the children. *J Epidemiol Comm Health* 35:155–160.

Bergen, D., C. M. Tanner, and R. Wilson (1982). The electroencephalogram in Tourette syndrome. *Ann Neurol* 11:382–385.

Berman, A. (1971). The problem of assessing cerebral dominance and its relationship to intelligence. *Cortex* 7:372–386.

Biegon, A., and B. S. McEwen (1982). Modulation by estradiol of serotonin receptors in brain. *J Neurosci* 2:199–205.

Bird, E. D., S. A. Chiappa, and G. Fink (1976). Brain immunoreactive gonadotropin-releasing hormone in Huntington's chorea and in non-choreic subjects. *Nature* 260:536–538.

Birky, C. W. (1983). Relaxed cellular controls and organelle heredity. *Science* 222:466–475.

Bishop, D. V. M. (1983). How sinister is sinistrality? *JRCP (Lon)* 17:161–172.

Black, I. B., and J. Axelrod (1983). The regulation of some biochemical circadian rhythms. In *Biochemical Actions of Hormones*, G. Litwack, ed., 135–155. New York: Academic Press.

Bleier, W. J., and M. Ehteshami (1981). Ovulation following unilateral ovariectomy in the California leaf-nosed bat (Macrotus californicus). *J Reprod Fert* 63:181–183.

Bockman, D. E., and M. L. Kirby (1984). Dependence of thymus development on derivatives of the neural crest. *Science* 223:498–500.

Bogen, J. E., and H. W. Gordon (1971). Musical tests for functional lateralization with intracarotid ambarbital. *Nature* 230:524–525.

Boklage, C. E. (1981). On the distribution of nonrighthandedness among twins and their families. *Acta Genet Med Gemellol* 30:167–187.

Boklage, C. E. (1984). Twinning, handedness and the biology of symmetry. In Geschwind and Galaburda, eds. (1984), 195–210.

Bongiovanni, A. M., A. M. Di George, and M. M. Grumbach (1959). Masculinization of the female infant associated with estrogenic therapy alone during gestation: Four cases. *J Clin Endocr* 19:1004–1011.

Bonin, G. von (1962). Anatomical asymmetries of the cerebral hemispheres. In *Interhemispheric Relations and Cerebral Dominance*. V. B. Mountcastle, ed., 1–6. Baltimore, Md.: The Johns Hopkins Press.

Boucher, J. (1977). Hand preference in autistic children and their parents. *J Autism Childhood Schiz* 7:177–187.

Boycott, A. E., and C. Diver (1923–24). On the inheritance of sinistrality in *Limnea peregra*. *Proc R Soc Lond* [Biol] 95:207–213.

Boycott, A. E., C. Diver, S. L. Garstang, et al. (1930). The inheritance of sinistrality in *Limnea peregra* (Mollusca, pulmonata). *Phil Trans Roy Soc Lond* Ser B, 219:51–131.

Bracco, L., A. Tiezzi, A. Ginanneschi, et al. (1984). Lateralization of choline acetyltransferase (ChAT) activity in fetus and adult human brain. *Neurosci Lett* 50:301–305.

Braitenberg, V., and M. Kemali (1970). Exceptions to bilateral symmetry in the epithalamus of lower vertebrates. *J Comp Neurol* 138:137–146.

Bray, P. F., and W. C. Wiser (1964). Evidence for a genetic etiology of temporal-central abnormalities in focal epilepsy. *NEJM* 271:926–933.

Bray, P. F., and W. C. Wiser (1965). The relation of focal to diffuse epileptiform EEG discharges in genetic epilepsy. *Arch Neurol* 13:223–237.

Bray, P. F., and W. C. Wiser (1969). A unifying concept of idiopathic epilepsy. *Postgrad Med* 46:82–87.

Breedlove, S. M., and A. P. Arnold (1980). Hormone accumulation in a sexually dimorphic motor nucleus of the rat spinal cord. *Science* 210:564–568.

Broca, P. (1861). Remarques sur le siège de la faculté du langage articulé, suivies d'une observation d'aphémie. *Bull Soc Anat Paris*, 2nd series, 6:398–407.

Broca, P. (1863). Localisation des fonctions cérébrales, siège de la faculté du langage articulé. *Bull Soc d'Anthropol Paris* 4:200–204.

Bronson, F. H., and C. Desjardins (1968). Aggression in adult mice: Modification by neonatal injections of gonadal hormones. *Science* 161:705–706.

Brumback, R. A., and R. D. Staton (1983). Learning disability and childhood depression. *Am J Orthopsychiatry* 53:269–281.

Bryden, M. P. (1982). *Laterality: Functional Asymmetry in the Intact Brain*. New York: Academic Press.

Buffery, A. W. H., and J. A. Gray (1972). Sex differences in the development of spatial and linguistic skills. In *Gender Differences: Their Ontogeny and Significance*, C. Ounsted and D. C. Taylor, eds. London: Churchill Livingstone.

Bulmer, M. G. (1970). *The Biology of Twinning in Man*. Oxford: Clarendon Press.

Burwell, R. G., P. H. Dangerfield, D. J. Hall, et al. (1978). Perthes' disease. *J Bone Joint Surg* 60B:461–477.

Byrne, B. (1974). Handedness and musical ability. *Br J Psychol* 65:279–281.

Cain, D. P., and J. A. Wada (1979). An anatomical asymmetry in the baboon brain. *Brain Behav Evol* 16:222–226.

Campain, R., and J. Minckler (1976). A note on the gross configurations of the human auditory cortex. *Brain Lang* 3:318–323.

Cappa, S. F., and L. A. Vignolo (1979). "Transcortical" features of aphasia following left thalamic hemorrhage. *Cortex* 15:121–130.

Caron, J.-P., H. Colin, J. Comoy, et al. (1982). Résultats de l'exérèse chirurgicale des aneurysmes artério-veineux (AAV) des zones rolandique, pariétale, occipitale, et du pli courbe de l'hémisphère dominant. À propos de vingt cas. *Neurochirurgie* 28:295–307.

Carpenter, S., R. Yassa, and R. Ochs (1982). A pathologic basis for Kleine-Levin syndrome. *Arch Neurol* 39:25–28.

Carter, C. O. (1972). Sex-linkage and sex-limitation. In *Gender Differences: Their Ontogeny and Significance.* C. Ounsted and D. C. Taylor, eds. London: Churchill Livingstone.

Castro, J. E. (1974). Orchidectomy and the immune response. I. Effect of orchidectomy on lymphoid tissues of mice. *Proc R Soc Lond* [Biol] 185:425–436.

Chang, K. S. F., F. K. Hsu, S. T. Chan, et al. (1960). Scrotal asymmetry and handedness. *J Anat* 94:543–548.

Channick, B. J., E. V. Adlin, A. D. Marks, et al. (1981). Hyperthyroidism and mitral-valve prolapse. *NEJM* 305:497–500.

Chesselett, M. F., N. Cheramy, T. D. Reisine, et al. (1983). Local and distal effects induced by unilateral striatal application of opiates in the absence or presence of naloxone on the release of dopamine in both caudate nuclei and substantiae nigrae of the cat. *Brain Res* 258:229–242.

Chhibber, S. R., and I. Singh (1970). Asymmetry in muscle weight and one-sided dominance in the human lower limbs. *J Anat* 106:553–556.

Chhibber, S. R., and I. Singh (1972). Asymmetry in the muscle weight in the human upper limbs. *Acta Anat* 81:462–465.

Chi, J. G., E. C. Dooling, and F. H. Gilles (1977). Left-right asymmetries of the temporal speech areas of the human fetus. *Arch Neurol* 34:346–348.

Chui, H. C., and A. R. Damasio (1980). Human cerebral asymmetries evaluated by computed tomography. *J Neurol Neurosurg Psychiatry* 43:873–878.

Chung, C. S., and N. C. Myrianthopoulos (1975). Factors affecting risks of congenital malformations. *Birth Defects* 11:23–38.

Churchill, J. A., E. Igna, and R. Seirf (1962). The association of position at birth and handedness. *Ped* 29:307–309.

Ciemins, V. A. (1970). Localized thalamic hemorrhage: A cause of aphasia. *Neurology* 20:776–782.

Cilluffo, J. M., M. R. Gomez, D. F. Reese, et al. (1981). Idiopathic ("congenital") spinal arachnoid diverticula. *Mayo Clin Proc* 56:93–101.

Clark, W. E. Le Gros (1927). Description of the cerebral hemispheres of a gorilla (John Daniels II). *J Anat* 61:467–475.

Claustrat, B., G. Chazot, J. Brun, et al. (1984). A chronobiological study of melatonin and cortisol secretion in depressed subjects: Plasma melatonin, a biochemical marker in major depression. *Biol Psychiatry* 14:1215–1228.

Clutton-Brock, T. H. (1982). Sons and daughters. *Nature* 298:11–13.

Cobb, S. (1915) Haemangioma of the spinal cord. *Ann Surgery* 62:641–649.

Colby, K. M., and C. Parkinson (1977). Handedness in autistic children. *J Autism Childhood Schiz* 7:3–9.

Coleman, M. (1976). *The Autistic Syndromes.* Amsterdam: North-Holland.

Collins, R. L. (1969). On the inheritance of handedness. 2. Selection for sinistrality in mice. *J Hered* 60:117–119.

Corballis, M. C., and M. J. Morgan (1978). On the biological basis of human laterality. *Behav Brain Sci* 2:261–336.

Coursey, R. D., M. S. Buchsbaum, and D. L. Murphy (1979). Platelet-MAO activity and evoked potentials in the identification of subjects biologically at risk for psychiatric disorders. *Br J Psychiatry* 134:372–381.

Cowan, W. M. (1973). Neuronal death as a regulative mechanism in the control of cell numbers in the nervous system. In *Development and Aging in the Nervous System,* M. Rockstein, ed., 19–41. New York: Academic Press.

Crawford, W. A., and C. G. Beldham (1976). The changing demographic pattern in asthma related to sex and age. *Med J Aust* 1:430–434.

Crosby, C. C., T. Humphrey, and E. W. Lauer (1962). *Correlative Anatomy of the Nervous System.* New York: Macmillan.

Crystal, H. A., D. S. Haroupian, R. Katzman, et al. (1982). Biopsy-proved Alzheimer disease presenting as a right parietal lobe syndrome. *Ann Neurol* 12:156–188.

Cummins, H., and C. Midlo (1943). *Finger Prints, Palms and Soles.* Philadelphia: The Blakeston Company.

Cunningham, D. J. (1892). *Contribution to the Surface Anatomy of the Cerebral Hemispheres.* Dublin: Royal Irish Academy.

Curry, J., and L. M. Heim (1966). Brain myelination after neonatal administration of oestradiol. *Nature* 209:915–916.

Cushing, H. (1906). Cases of spontaneous intracranial hemorrhage associated with trigeminal nevi. *JAMA* 47:178–183.

Cynader, M., F. Lepore, and J.-P. Guillemot (1981). Interhemispheric competition during postnatal development. *Nature* 290:139–140.

Dahlberg, G. (1944–47). Genotypic asymmetries. *Proc R Soc Edin*, Sect B, 62:20–31.

Dalby, M. A. (1981). Attentional difficulties and subclinical absences in specific language delayed children. *Abstracts, World Congress of Neurology*, Kyoto, 118. Int. Congress Series 548. Amsterdam: Excerpta Medica.

Davidson, E. H., B. R. Hough-Evans, and R. J. Britten (1982). Molecular biology of the sea urchin embryo. *Science* 217:17–26.

Davis, M. R., M. Constantine-Paton, and D. Schorr (1983). Dorsal root ganglion removal in *Rana pipieus* produces fewer motoneurones. *Brain Res* 265:283–288.

DeBassio, W. A., and T. L. Kemper (1982). Neuronal migration in undernourished rats. *Ann Neurol* 12:222.

DeBassio, W. A., T. L. Kemper, and A. M. Galaburda (1982). Asymmetric olfactory migratory stream growth in the rat. *Soc Neurosci Abstr* 8:326.

Déjerine, J. (1891). Sur un cas de cécité verbale avec agraphie, suivi d'autopsie. *Mem Soc Biol* 3:197–201.

Denef, C. (1976). Differentiation of steroid metabolism in the rat and mechanisms of neonatal androgen action. *Enzyme* 15:254–271.

Denef, C., and P. DeMoor (1968). The "puberty" of the rat liver. II. Permanent changes in steroid metabolizing enzymes after treatment with a single injection of testosterone proprionate at birth. *Endocrinology* 83:791–798.

Denenberg, V. H. (1981). Hemispheric laterality in animals and the effects of early experience. *Behav Brain Sci* 4:1–49.

Denenberg, V. H., J. Garbanati, G. Sherman, et al. (1978). Infantile stimulation induces brain lateralization in rats. *Science* 201:1150–1152.

Denenberg, V. H., and M. X. Zarrow (1971). Effects of handling in infancy upon adult behavior and adrenocortical activity: Suggestions for a neuroendocrine mechanism. In *The Development of Self-Regulatory Mechanisms*, D. N. Walcher and D. L. Peters, eds., 39–64. New York: Academic Press.

Deutsch, D. (1978). Pitch memory: An advantage for the lefthanded. *Science* 199:559–560.

Devereux, R. B., W. T. Brown, E. M. Lutas, et al. (1982). Association of mitral-valve prolapse with low body-weight and low blood pressure. *Lancet* 2:792–794.

Dewson, J. H., III (1979). Toward an animal model of auditory cognitive function. In *The Neurological Bases of Language Disorders in Children: Methods and Directions for Research*, C. L. Ludlow and M. E. Doran-Quine, eds., 19–24. NINCDS Monograph No. 22. Washington, D.C.: Government Printing Office.

Diamond, M. C. (1984). Age, sex, and environmental influences. In Geschwind and Galaburda, eds. (1984), 134–146.

Diamond, M. C., G. A. Dowling, and R. E. Johnson (1981). Morphological cerebral cortical asymmetry in male and female rats. *Exp Neurol* 71:261–268.

Diamond, M. C., R. E. Johnson, and C. A. Ingham (1975). Morphological changes in the young, adult and aging rat cerebral cortex, hippocampus and diencephalon. *Behav Biol* 14:163–174.

Diamond, M. C., R. E. Johnson, D. Young, et al. (1983). Age related morphologic differences in the rat cerebral cortex and hippocampus: Male-female; right-left. *Exp Neurol* 81:1–13.

Diamond, M. C., G. M. Murphy, Jr., K. Akiama, et al. (1982). Morphologic hippocampal asymmetry in male and female rats. *Exp Neurol* 76:553–565.

Diehl, C. F. (1958). *A Compendium of Research and Theory on Stuttering.* Springfield, Ill.: Charles C. Thomas.

DiPaolo, G. A. (1964). Polydactylism in the offspring of mice injected with 5-bromodoxyuridine. *Science* 145:501–503.

Dohler, K. D. (1978). Is female sexual differentiation hormone-mediated? *TINS* 1:138–140.

Dörner, G. (1980). Sexual differentiation of the brain. *Vitamins and Hormones* 38:325–381.

Dörner, G., F. Gotz, and W.-D. Docke (1983). Prevention of demasculinization and feminization of the brain in prenatally stressed male rats by perinatal androgen treatment. *Exper Clin Endocrinol* 81:88–90.

Dörner, G., B. Schenk, B. Schmiedel, et al. (1983). Stressful events in prenatal life of bi- and homosexual men. *Exper Clin Endocrinol* 81:83–87.

Dougherty, T. F. (1952). Effects of hormones on lymphatic tissue. *Physiol Rev* 32:379–401.

Drake, W. E. (1968). Clinical and pathological findings in a child with a developmental learning disability. *J Learn Disabil* 1:9–25.

Draper, G., C. W. Dupertuis, and J. L. Caughey, Jr. (1944). *Human Constitution in Clinical Medicine.* New York: Paul B. Hoeber.

Dunn, L. C. (1964). Abnormalities associated with a chromosome region in the mouse. *Science* 144:260–267.

Durfee, K. E. (1974). Crooked ears and the bad boy syndrome: Asymmetry as an indicator of minimal brain dysfunction. *Bull Menninger Clin* 38:305–316.

Duvoisin, R. C., R. Eldridge, A. Williams, et al. (1981). Twin study of Parkinson disease. *Neurology* 31:77–80.

Eberstaller, O. (1884). Zur oberflächen Anatomie des Grosshirn Hemisphären. *Wien Med Blätter* 7:479, 642, 644.

Economo, C. von, and L. Horn (1930). Über Windungsrelief, Masse und Rindenarchitektonik der Supratemporalfläche, ihre individuellen und ihre Seitenunterschiede. *Ztschr Ges Neurol Psychiat* 130:678–757.

Edwards, D. A. (1964). Mice: Fighting by neonatally androgenized females. *Science* 161:1027–1028.

Egger, J., C. M. Carter, J. Wilson, et al. (1983). Is migraine food allergy? *Lancet* 2:865–870.

Ehrhardt, A. A., and J. Money (1967). Progestin-induced hermaphroditism: IQ and psychosexual identity in a study of ten girls. *J Sex Res* 3:83–100.

Eidelberg, D., and A. M. Galaburda (1982). Symmetry and asymmetry in the human posterior thalamus. I. Cytoarchitectonic analysis in normal persons. *Arch Neurol* 39:325–332.

Eidelberg, D., and A. M. Galaburda (1984). Inferior parietal lobule: Divergent architectonic asymmetries in the human brain. *Arch Neurol* 41:843–852.

Engbretson, G. A., A. Reiner, and N. Brecha (1981). Habenular asymmetry and the central connections of the parietal eye of the lizard. *J Comp Neurol* 198:155–165.

Epstein, E. (1971). Triamcinolone-procaine in the treatment of zoster and postzoster neuralgia. *Calif Med* 115:6–10.

Esscher, E., and J. S. Scott (1979). Congenital heart block and maternal systemic lupus erythematosus. *Br Med J* 1:1235–1238.

Faden, A. I., T. P. Jacobs, M. Woods, et al. (1978). Zona intermedia pressor sites in the cat spinal cord: Right-left asymmetry. *Exp Neurol* 61:571–582.

Falconer, M. A., and W. A. Kennedy (1961). Epilepsy due to small focal temporal lesions with bilateral independent spike-discharging foci: A study of seven cases relieved by operation. *J Neurol Neurosurg Psychiatry* 24:205–212.

Falzi, G., P. Perrone, and L. A. Vignolo (1982). Right-left asymmetry in anterior speech region. *Arch Neurol* 39:239–240.

Faris, R. A., and T. C. Campbell (1981). Exposure of newborn rats to pharmacologically active compounds may permanently alter carcinogen metabolism. *Science* 211:719–721.

Farthing, M. J. G., C. R. W. Edwards, L. H. Rees, et al. (1982). Male gonadal function in coeliac disease: 1. Sexual dysfunction, infertility, and semen quality. *Gut* 23:608–614.

Faulk, W. P. (1981). Human trophoblast antigens. Role in normal and abnormal pregnancies. *Bull Mém l'Acad royale Méd Bel* (Bulletin et Mémoires de l'Académie royale de Médecine de Belgique) 136:379–388.

Fialkow, P. J. (1964). Autoimmunity: A predisposing factor to chromosomal aberrations? *Lancet* 1:474–475.

Fialkow, P. J. (1970). Thyroid autoimmunity and Down's syndrome. *Ann NY Acad Sci* 171:500–511.

Fischer, E. (1921). Ueber die Variationen der Hirnfurchen des Schimpansen. *Verh Anat Ges (Jena)* 30:48–54.

Flanders, M., and D. Swann (1977). *The Songs of Michael Flanders and Donald Swann.* New York: St. Martin's Press.

Flechsig, P. (1876). *Die Leitungsbahnen in Gehirn und Rückenmark des Menschen auf Grund entwicklungsgeschichtlicher Untersuchungen.* Leipzig: W. Engelmann.

Folstein, S., and M. Rutter (1977). Genetic influences and infantile autism. *Nature* 265:726–728.

Fontes, V. (1944). *Morfologia do Cortex Cerebral (Desenvolvimento).* Lisbon: Instituto Antonio Aurelio da Costa Ferreira.

Fraser, F. C. (1983). Association of neural tube defects and parental non-righthandedness. *Am J Human Gen* 35:89A.

Fraser, F. C., A. Czeizel, and C. Hanson (1982). Increased frequency of neural tube defects in sibs of children with other malformations. *Lancet* 2:144–145.

Freeman, G., and J. W. Lundelius (1982). The developmental genetics of dextrality and sinistrality in the gastropod *Lymnea peregra. W Roux's Arch* 191:69–83.

Freeman, R. L., A. M. Galaburda, R. Díaz-Cabal, et al. (1985). The neurology of depression: Cognitive and behavioral deficits with focal findings in depression and resolution after electroconvulsive therapy. *Arch Neurol* 42:289–291.

Frey-Wettstein, M., and C. G. Craddock (1970). Testosterone-induced depletion of thymus and marrow lymphocytes as related to lymphopoiesis and hematopoiesis. *Blood* 35:257–271.

Fukui, T. (1934). Transverse gyri of temporal lobe in the Japanese brain, 5th report. *Hokuetsu Igaku Zasshi* 49:1025–1050.

Furukawa, T., and T. Shinohara (1981). Congenital hemihypertrophy: Oncogenic potential of the hypertrophic side. *Ann Neurol* 10:199–201.

Gabrielli, W. F., and S. A. Mednick (1983). Intellectual performance in children of alcoholics. *J Nerv Ment Dis* 171:444–447.

Gainotti, G. (1972). Emotional behavior and hemispheric side of the lesion. *Cortex* 8:41–55.

Galaburda, A. M. (1980). La région de Broca: Observations anatomiques faites un siècle après la mort de son découvreur. *Rev Neurol (Paris)* 136, 10:609–616.

Galaburda, A. M. (1983). Developmental dyslexia: Current anatomical research. *Ann Dyslexia* 33:41–53.

Galaburda, A. M. (1984). Anatomical asymmetries. In Geschwind and Galaburda, eds. (1984), 11–25.

Galaburda, A. M., and D. Eidelberg (1982). Symmetry and asymmetry in the human posterior thalamus. Part II: Thalamic lesions in a case of developmental dyslexia. *Arch Neurol* 39:333–336.

Galaburda, A. M., and T. L. Kemper (1979). Cytoarchitectonic abnormalities in developmental dyslexia: A case study. *Ann Neurol* 6:94–100.

Galaburda, A. M., M. Le May, T. L. Kemper, et al. (1978). Right-left asymmetries in the brain. *Science* 199:852–856.

Galaburda, A. M., and F. Sanides (1980). Cytoarchitectonic organization of the human auditory cortex. *J Comp Neurol* 190:597–610.

Galaburda, A. M., F. Sanides, and N. Geschwind (1978). Human brain: Cytoarchitectonic left-right asymmetries in the temporal speech region. *Arch Neurol* 35:812–817.

Galaburda, A. M., G. F. Sherman, G. D. Rosen, et al. (1985). Developmental dyslexia: Four consecutive cases with cortical anomalies. *Ann Neurol* 18:222–233.

Gandelman, R., F. S. vom Saal, and J. M. Reinisch (1977). Contiguity to male foetuses affects morphology and behaviour of female mice. *Nature* 266:722–725.

Garay, A. S. (1968). Origin and role of optical isomery in life. *Nature* 219:338–340.

Gathier, J. C., and G. W. Bruyn (1970a). Neuralgic amyopathy. In *Handbook of Clinical Neurology*. Vol. 8: *Diseases of Nerves, Part II*, P. J. Vinken and G. W. Bruyn, eds., 77–85. New York: American Elsevier.

Gathier, J. C., and G. W. Bruyn (1970b). The serogenetic peripheral neuropathies. In *Handbook of Clinical Neurology*. Vol. 8: *Diseases of Nerves, Part II*, P. J. Vinken and G. W. Bruyn, eds., 95–111. New York: American Elsevier.

Gentili, C., and F. Tiberi (1963). Rilievi clinico-sperimentali sull'azione neuropsicodislettica della N-N-dietiltriptamina. *Atti del 2° Colloquio Internazionale sull'Espressione Plastica*, Bologna.

Gerendai, I. (1984). Lateralization of neuroendocrine control. In Geschwind and Galaburda, eds. (1984), 167–178.

Gerendai, I., W. Rosztejn, B. Marchetti, et al. (1978). Unilateral ovariectomy-induced luteinizing hormone-releasing hormone content changes in the two halves of the mediobasal hypothalamus. *Neurosci Lett* 9:333–336.

Geschwind, N. (1975). The apraxias: Neural mechanisms of disorders of learned movement. *American Scientist* 63:188–195.

Geschwind, N. (1983). Pathogenesis of behavior changes in temporal lobe epilepsy. In *Epilepsy*, A. A. Ward, Jr., J. K. Penry, and D. Purpura, eds., 355–370. New York: Raven Press.

Geschwind, N., and P. Behan (1982). Left-handedness: Association with immune disease, migraine, and developmental learning disorder. *Proc Natl Acad Sci USA* 79:5097–5100.

Geschwind, N., and P. Behan (1984). Laterality, hormones and immunity. In Geschwind and Galaburda, eds. (1984), 211–224.

Geschwind, N., and A. M. Galaburda, eds. (1984). *Cerebral Dominance: The Biological Foundations.* Cambridge, Mass.: Harvard University Press.

Geschwind, N., and W. Levitsky (1968). Human brain: Left-right asymmetries in temporal speech region. *Science* 161:186–187.

Gesell, A. (1927). Hemihypertrophy and twinning. *Am J Sci* 173:542–555.

Gesell, A., and L. B. Ames (1947). The development of handedness. *J Genet Psychol* 70:155–175.

Ghosh, A., J. S. K. Woo, I. M. L. Poon, et al. (1981). Neural tube defects in Hong Kong Chinese. *Lancet* 2:468–469.

Giron, L. T., Jr., K. A. Crutcher, and J. N. Davis (1980). Lymph nodes: A possible site for sympathetic neuronal regulation of immune responses. *Ann Neurol* 8:520–525.

Glick, S. D. (1983). Heritable determinants of left-right bias in the rat. *Life Sci* 32:2215–2221.

Glick, S. D., ed. (1985). *Cerebral Lateralization in Nonhuman Species.* New York: Academic Press.

Glick, S. D., and R. D. Cox (1978). Nocturnal rotation in normal rats: Correlation with amphetamine-induced rotation and effects of nigrostriatal lesions. *Brain Res* 150:149–161.

Glick, S. D., T. P. Jerussi, and L. N. Fleisher (1976). Turning in circles: The neuropharmacology of rotation. *Life Sci* 18:889–896.

Glick, S. D., T. P. Jerussi, P. H. Waters, et al. (1974). Amphetamine-induced changes in striatal dopamine and acetylcholine levels and relationship to rotation (circling behavior) in rats. *Biochem Pharmacol* 23:3223–3225.

Glick, S. D., R. C. Meibach, R. D. Cox, et al. (1979). Multiple and interrelated functional asymmetries in rat brain. *Life Sci* 25:395–400.

Glick, S. D., D. A. Ross, and L. B. Hough (1982). Lateral asymmetry of neurotransmitters in human brain. *Brain Res* 234:53–63.

Glick, S., and R. Shapiro (1984). Functional and neurochemical asymmetries. In Geschwind and Galaburda, eds. (1984), 147–166.

Gloning, I., K. Gloning, G. Haub, et al. (1969). Comparison of verbal behavior in right-handed and non right-handed patients with anatomically verified lesion of one hemisphere. *Cortex* 5:43–52.

Goldman, P. S. (1978). Neuronal plasticity in primate telencephalon: Anomalous projections induced by prenatal removal of frontal cortex. *Science* 202:768–770.

Goldman, P. S. (1979). Contralateral projections to the dorsal thalamus from frontal association cortex in the rhesus monkey. *Brain Res* 166:166–171.

Goldman, P. S., and T. W. Galkin (1978). Prenatal removal of frontal association cortex in the fetal rhesus monkey: Anatomical and functional consequences in postnatal life. *Brain Res* 152:451–485.

Goldman-Rakic, P., and P. Rakic (1984). Experimental modification of gyral patterns. In Geschwind and Galaburda, eds. (1984), 179–192.

Golub, E. S. (1982). Connections between the neurons, haematopoietic and germ-cell systems. *Nature* 299:483–485.

Goodall, H. B., and G. W. Brobby (1982). Stuttering, sickling and cerebral malaria: A possible organic basis for stuttering. *Lancet* 1:1279–1281.

Goodfellow, P. N., and P. W. Andrews (1983). Is there a human T/t locus? *Nature* 302:657–658.

Goodglass, H., and F. A. Quadfasel (1954). Language laterality in left-handed aphasics. *Brain* 77:521–548.

Gordon, H. W. (1980). Cognitive asymmetry in dyslexic families. *Neuropsychologia* 18:645–656.

Gordon, H. W. (1983). Learning disabled are cognitively right. In *Topics in Learning Disabilities*, vol. 3, M. Kinsbourne, ed., 29–39. Rockville, Md.: Aspen Systems Corp.

Gorski, R. A., R. E. Harlan, C. D. Jacobson, et al. (1980). Evidence for the existence of a sexually dimorphic nucleus in the preoptic area of the rat. *J Comp Neurol* 193:529–539.

Govind, C. K., and K. S. Kent (1982). Transformation of fast fibres to slow prevented by lack of activity in developing lobster muscle. *Nature* 298:755–757.

Govind, C. K., and R. E. Young (1983). Lateralization of the nervous system to the paired asymmetric chelipedes of male fiddler crabs. *Soc Neurosci Abstr* 9:383.

Graff-Radford, N. R., P. J. Eslinger, A. R. Damasio, et al. (1984). Nonhemorrhagic infarction of the thalamus: Behavioral, anatomic, and physiologic correlates. *Neurology* 34:14–23.

Graham, J. R., A. Z. Rogado, M. Rahman, et al. (1970). Some physical, physiological and psychological characteristics of patients with cluster headaches. In *Background to Migraine: Third Migraine Symposium*, A. L. Cochrane, ed. New York: Springer-Verlag.

Grapin, P., and C. Perpère (1968). Symétrie et latéralisation du nourrisson. In *Main droite et main gauche*, R. Kourilsky and P. Grapin, eds., 83–100. Paris: Presses Universitaires de France.

Greenfield, J. G., W. Blackwood, W. H. McMenemy, et al., eds. (1958). *Neuropathology*. London: Edward Arnold.

Groves, C. P., and N. K. Humphrey (1973). Asymmetry in gorilla skulls: Evidence of lateralized brain function? *Nature* 244:53–54.

Gruzellier, J., and P. Flor-Henry (1979). *Hemispheric Asymmetries of Function in Psychopathology*. Amsterdam: Elsevier/North-Holland Biomedical Press.

Gundara, N., and B. Zivanovic (1968). Asymmetry in East African skulls. *Amer J Phys Anthrop* 28:331–338.

Gupta, C., S. J. Yaffee, and B. H. Shapiro (1982). Prenatal exposure to phenobarbital permanently decreases testosterone and causes reproductive dysfunction. *Science* 216:640–642.

Gustaffson, J.-A., A. Mode, P. Skett, et al. (1978). Cerebral control of a cytochrome P-450-dependent steroid hydroxylase in rat liver. In *Hormones and Brain Development*, C. Dorner and M. Kawakami, eds., 139–146. Amsterdam: Elsevier/North-Holland Biomedical Press.

Haagensen, C. D. (1971). *Diseases of the Breast*. 2nd ed. Philadelphia: W. B. Saunders Co.

Hall, J. G., J. Levin, J. P. Kuhn, et al. (1969). Thrombocytopenia with absent radius (TAR). *Medicine (Baltimore)* 48:411–439.

Hamburger, V., and R. W. Oppenheim (1982). Naturally occurring neuronal death in vertebrates. *Neurosci Commentaries* 1:39–55.

Hamlin, R. M. (1970). Intellectual function 14 years after frontal lobe surgery. *Cortex* 6:299–307.

Harati, Y., J. S. Meyer, and A. H. Wheeler (1981). Neuroanatomical and neurophysiological explanations for mirror movement in Klippel-Feil syndrome derived from rcBF studies. *Abstracts, World Congress of Neurology*, Kyoto, 386. Int. Congress Series 548. Amsterdam: Excerpta Medica.

Harper, P. S. (1979). *Myotonic Dystrophy*. Philadelphia: W. B. Saunders Co.

Harvey, P. H., and M. Slatkin (1982). Some like it hot: Temperature-determined sex. *Nature* 296:807–808.

Haseltine, F. P., and S. Ohno (1981). Mechanisms of gonadal differentiation. *Science* 211:1272–1278.

Hauser, H., and R. Gandelman (1983). Contiguity to males in utero affects avoidance responding in adult female mice. *Science* 220:437–438.

Heacock, A. M., and B. W. Agranoff (1977). Clockwise growth of neurites from retinal explants. *Science* 198:64–66.

Hecaen, H. (1984). *Les gauchers*. Paris: Presses Universitaires de France.

Hecaen, H., and J. de Ajuriaguerra (1964). *Left-Handedness*. New York: Grune and Stratton.

Heilman, K. M., H. Schwartz, and R. T. Watson (1977). Hypoarousal in patients with the neglect syndrome and emotional indifference. *Neurology* 28:229–232.

Heim, L. M., and P. S. Timiras (1963). Gonad-brain relationship: Precocious brain maturation after estradiol in rats. *Endocrinology* 72:598–606.

Heinonen, D. P., D. Slone, R. R. Monson, et al. (1977). Cardiovascular birth defects and antenatal exposure to female sex hormones. *NEJM* 296:67–70.

Henschen, S. E. (1926). On the function of the right hemisphere of the brain in relation to the left in speech, music and calculation. *Brain* 49:110–123.

Herbst, A. L., M. M. Hubby, R. R. Blough, et al. (1980). A comparison of pregnancy experience in DES-exposed and DES-unexposed daughters. *J Reprod Med* 24:62–69.

Hermann, K. (1959). *Reading Disability*. Springfield, Ill.: Charles C. Thomas.

Hervé, G. (1888). *La circonvolution de Broca*. Paris: Delahage et Lecrosnier.

Herzog, A. G., V. Russell, J. L. Vaitukaitis, et al. (1982). Neuroendocrine dysfunction in temporal lobe epilepsy. *Arch Neurol* 39:133–135.

Herzog, A. G., M. M. Seibel, D. Schomer, et al. (1984). Temporal lobe epilepsy: An extrahypothalamic pathogenesis for polycystic ovarian syndrome? *Neurology* 34:1389–1393.

Heydemann, P. T., and P. R. Huttenlocher (1982). Synaptogenesis, synaptic density, and the effect of cortisol in reaggregated mouse cerebral isocortex: A model for evaluating drug effects on synaptic movement. *Ann Neurol* 12:202.

Hicks, R. E., and A. K. Barton (1975). A note on left-handedness and severity of mental retardation. *J Genet Psychol* 127:323–324.

Hier, D. B., and W. F. Crowley, Jr. (1982). Spatial ability in androgen-deficient men. *NEJM* 306:1202–1205.

Hier, D. B., M. LeMay, and P. B. Rosenberger (1979). Developmental dyslexia and unfavorable left-right asymmetries of the brain. *J Autism and Dev Dis* 9:153–159.

Hier, D. B., M. LeMay, P. B. Rosenberger, et al. (1978). Developmental dyslexia: Evidence for a sub-group with reversed cerebral asymmetry. *Arch Neurol* 35:90–92.

Hines, M. (1982). Prenatal gonadal hormones and sex differences in human behavior. *Psychol Bull* 92:56–80.

Hochberg, F. M., and M. LeMay (1975). Arteriographic correlates of handedness. *Neurology* 25:218–222.

Holloway, R. L. (1980). Indonesian "Solo" (Ngadong) endocranial reconstructions: Some preliminary observations and comparisons with Neanderthal and Homo erectus groups. *Amer J Phys Anthrop* 53:285–295.

Holloway, R. J., and C. de Lacoste (1982). Brain endocast asymmetry in pongids and hominlids: The paleontology of cerebral hemisphere dominance. *Amer J Phys Anthrop* 58:101–110.

Honzik, M. P., D. S. Collart, S. J. Robinson, et al. (1969). Sex differences in verbal and performance IQ's of children undergoing open-heart surgery. *Science* 164:445–447.

Howard, J., N. L. Petrakis, I. D. Bross, et al. (1982). Handedness and breast cancer laterality: Testing a hypothesis. *Human Biol* 54:365–371.

Hunt, J. R. (1917). Progressive atrophy of the globus pallidus (primary atrophy of pallidal system): A system disease of paralysis agitans type. *Brain* 40:58–148.

Huppert, L. C. (1979). Induction of ovulation with clomiphene citrate. *Modern Trends* 31:1–8.

Huttenlocher, P. R. (1979). Synaptic density in the human frontal cortex: Developmental changes and effects of aging. *Brain Res* 163:195–205.

Ingalls, N. W. (1914). The parietal region in the primate brain. *J Comp Neurol* 28:291–341.

Innocenti, G. M. (1981). Growth and reshaping of axons in the establishment of visual callosal connections. *Science* 212:824–827.

Ivanyi, P. (1978). Some aspects of the H-2 system, the major histocompatibility system in the mouse. *Proc R Soc Lond* [Biol] 202:117–158.

Jacob, J. C., F. Andermann, and J. P. Robb (1961). Heredofamilial neuritis with brachial predilection. *Neurology* 11:1025–1033.

Jacobson, C.-O. (1959). The localization of the presumptive cerebral regions in the neural plate of the axolate larva. *J Embryol Exp Morphol* 7:1–21.

Jacobson, M. (1978). *Developmental Neurobiology.* New York: Plenum Press.

Jaffee, W. L., and J. L. Vaitukaitis (1982). Polycystic ovarian syndrome. In *Clinical and Reproductive Neuroendocrinology,* J. L. Vaitukaitis, ed., 207–230. New York: Elsevier.

James, W. H. (1980a). Gonadotrophin and the human secondary sex ratio. *Br Med J* 281:711–712.

James, W. H. (1980b). Race, season, gonadotrophin, and sex ratio. *Lancet* 2:1032.

Janerich, D. T., J. M. Piper, and D. M. Glebatis (1974). Oral contraceptives and congenital limb-reduction defects. *NEJM* 291:697–700.

Jannetta, P. J. (1981). Vascular decompression in trigeminal neuralgia. In *The Cranial Nerves*, M. Samii and P. J. Jannetta, eds., 331–340. Berlin-New York: Springer-Verlag.

Jannetta, P. J., and H. M. Gendell (1979). Clinical observations on etiology of essential hypertension. *Surg Forum* 30:431–432.

Jenkins, J. B. (1979). *Genetics*. 2nd ed. Boston: Houghton Mifflin.

Jerussi, T. P., and S. D. Glick (1976). Drug-induced rotation in rats without lesions: Behavioral and neurochemical indices of a normal asymmetry in nigro-striatal function. *Psychopharmacology* 47:249–260.

Johnston, J. B. (1902). The brain of Petromyzon. *J Comp Neurol* 12:1–86.

Jovanovic, V. J. (1971). Physiologische Mykloni beim Einschlafen und im Schlaf. *Z EEG-EMG* 2:58–63.

Kakeshita, T. (1925). Zur Anatomie der operkularen Temporal-Region: Vergleichende Untersuchungen der rechten und linken Seite. *Arb Neurol Inst Wien* 27:292.

Kallen, B. (1967). *Teratology, The Science of Malformations*. Stockholm: Almquist and Wiksell.

Kappers, C. V. A., G. C. Huber, and E. C. Crosby (1936). *The Comparative Anatomy of the Nervous System of Vertebrates including Man*. New York: Macmillan.

Karfunkel, P. (1974). The mechanisms of neural tube formation. *Int Rev Cytol* 38:245–271.

Karsch, F. J., D. J. Dierschke, and E. Knobil (1973). Sexual differentiation of pituitary function: Apparent difference between primates and rodents. *Science* 179:484–486.

Keller, R. (1942). Two famous left-handers. *Ciba Symposia* 3:1143–1145.

Kemali, M., V. Guilielmotti, and D. Gioffre (1980). Neuroanatomical identification of the frog habenular connections using peroxidase (HRP). *Exp Brain Res* 38:341–347.

Kemper, T. L. (1984). Asymmetrical lesions in dyslexia. In Geschwind and Galaburda, eds. (1984), 75–89.

Kertesz, A., and N. Geschwind (1971). Patterns of pyramidal decussation and their relationship to handedness. *Arch Neurol* 24:326–332.

Kidd, K. K., R. C. Heimbuch, and M. A. Records (1981). Vertical transmission of susceptibility to stuttering with sex-modified expression. *Proc Natl Acad Sci USA* 78:606–610.

Kilshaw, D., and M. Annett (1983). Right- and left-hand skill I: Effects of age, sex and hand preference showing superior skill in left-handers. *Br J Psychol* 74:253–268.

Kimura, D., and Y. Archibald (1974). Motor functions of the left hemisphere. *Brain* 97:337–350.

King, L. S. (1936). Hereditary defects of the corpus callosum in the mouse, *Mus musculus. J Comp Neurol* 64:337–363.

Kinsbourne, M., and E. K. Warrington (1963). The developmental Gerstmann syndrome. *Arch Neurol* 8:490–501.

Kissebah, A. H., N. Vydeligum, R. Murray, et al. (1982). Relation of body fat distribution to metabolic complications of obesity. *J Clin Endocrinol Metab* 54:253–260.

Koike, K., A. K. Rao, H. Holmsen, et al. (1984). Platelet-secretion defect in patients with the atttention deficit disorder. *Blood* 63:427–433.

Kolata, G. (1983). Math genius may have hormonal basis. *Science* 222:1312.

Kolb, B., A. McIntosh, I. Q. Wishaw, et al. (1984). Evidence for an anatomical but not functional asymmetry in the hemidecorticate rat. *Behav Neurosci* 98:44–58.

Kolb, B., R. J. Sutherland, A. J. Nonneman, et al. (1982). Asymmetry in the cerebral hemispheres of the rat, mouse, rabbit and cat: The right hemisphere is larger. *Exp Neurol* 78:348–359.

Kolodny, E. (1984). A postulated role for neutral hydrolases in developing brain. *Discussions in Neurosciences* 1, 2:89–91.

Kopp, N., F. Michel, H. Carrier, et al. (1977). Étude de certaines asymétries hemisphériques du cerveau humain. *J Neurol Sci* 34:349–363.

Korein, J. (1981). Iris pigmentation (melanin) in idiopathic dystonic syndromes including torticollis. *Ann Neurol* 10:53–55.

Korein, J. (1982). Response to Lang et al. *Ann Neurol* 12:586.

Kudrow, L. (1974). Physical and personality characteristics in cluster headache. *Headache* 13:197–202.

Kuritzky, A., D. K. Ziegler, and R. Hassanein, (1981). Vertigo, motion sickness and migraine. *Headache* 21:227–231.

Lang, A. E., C. Ellis, H. Kingon, et al. (1982). Iris pigmentation in idiopathic dystonia. *Ann Neurol* 12:585–586.

Larrabee, A. P. (1906). The optic chiasm of teleosts: A study of inheritance. *Proc Amer Acad Arts & Sciences* 12:217–231.

Layton, W. M., Jr. (1976). Random determination of a developmental process. *J Hered* 67:336–338.

Layton, W. M., Jr., and D. W. Hallesy (1965). Deformity of forelimb in rats: Association with high doses of acetazolamide. *Science* 149:306–308.

LeDouarin, N. (1982). *The Neural Crest.* Cambridge: Cambridge University Press.

LeMarec B., M. Roussey, J. Oger, et al. (1978). Excess twinning in the parents of spina bifida. In *Twin Research: Biology and Epidemiology*, W. E. Nance, ed., 121–123. New York: A. R. Liss.

LeMay, M. (1976). Morphological cerebral asymmetries of modern man, fossil man, and non-human primate. *Ann NY Acad Sci* 280:349–366.

LeMay, M. (1977). Asymmetries of the skull and handedness. *J Neurol Sci* 32:243–253.

LeMay, M. (1984). Radiological, developmental, and fossil asymmetries. In Geschwind and Galaburda, eds. (1984), 26–42.

LeMay, M., and A. Culebras (1972). Human brain: Morphologic differences in the hemispheres demonstrable by carotid arteriography. *NEJM* 287:168–170.

LeMay, M., and N. Geschwind (1975). Hemispheric differences in the brains of great apes. *Brain Behav Evol* 11:48–52.

Leppick, I. (1985). Seasonal allergy to phenytoin not related to dose. *Ann Neurol* 42:120–122.

Levine, D. N., D. B. Hier, and R. Calvanio (1981). Acquired learning disability for reading after left temporal lobe damage in childhood. *Neurology* 31:257–264.

Levitt, P. (1984). A monoclonal antibody to limbic system neurons. *Science* 223:299–301.

Levy, E. P., A. Cohen, and F. C. Fraser (1973). Hormone treatment during pregnancy and congenital heart defects. *Lancet* 1:611.

Levy, J. (1974). Psychobiological implications of bilateral asymmetry. In *Hemisphere Function in the Human Brain*, S. J. Dimond and J. G. Beaumont, eds., 121–183. London: P. Elek.

Levy, J., and M. Reid (1976). Variations in working posture and cerebral organization. *Science* 194:337–339.

Liepmann, H. (1908). *Drei Aufsätze aus dem Apraxiegebiet*. Berlin: Karger.

Lishman, W. A., and E. R. L. McMeekan (1976). Hand preference patterns in psychiatric patients. *Br J Psychiatry* 129:158–166.

Liszka, D. (1961). Spinal cord mechanisms leading to scoliosis in animal experiments. *Acta Med Pol* 2:45–67.

Lorber, C. A., S. B. Cassidy, and E. Engel (1979). Is there an embryo-fetal exogenous sex steroid exposure syndrome (EFESSES)? *Fertil Steril* 31:21–24.

Ludlow, C. L., R. J. Polinsky, E. D. Caine, et al. (1982). Language and speech abnormalities in Tourette syndrome. In *Gilles de la Tourette Syndrome*, H. J. Friedhoff and T. N. Chase, eds., 351–361. New York: Raven Press.

Luria, A. R. (1970). *Traumatic Aphasia*. The Hague: Mouton.

Luria, A. R. (1977). On quasi-aphasic speech disturbances in lesions of the deep structures of the brain. *Brain Lang* 4:432–459.

McAllister, L. B., R. H. Scheller, E. R. Kandel, et al. (1983). In situ hyridization to study the origin and fate of identified neurons. *Science* 222:800–808.

Maccoby, E. M., and C. N. Jacklin (1974). *The Psychology of Sex Differences.* Stanford, Calif.: Stanford University Press.

McEwen, B. S. (1981). Neural gonadal steroid actions. *Science* 211:1303–1311.

MacEwen, G. D. (1972). Operative treatment of scoliosis in cerebral palsy. *Reconstr Surg Traumat* 13:58–67.

McGee, M. G., and T. Cozad (1980). Population genetic analysis of human hand preference: Evidence for generational differences, familial resemblance, and maternal effects. *Behav Genet* 10:263–275.

McLean, J. M., and F. M. Ciurczak (1982). Bimanual dexterity in major league baseball players: A statistical study. *NEJM* 2:1278–1279.

MacLusky, N. J., and F. Naftolin (1981). Sexual differentiation of the central nervous system. *Science* 211:1294–1303.

McNeil, T. E., and L. Kaij (1978). Obstetric factors in the development of schizophrenia: Complications in the births of preschizophrenics and in reproduction by schizophrenic parents. In *The Nature of Schizophrenia,* L. C. Wynne, R. L. Cromwell, and S. Matthysse, eds., 401–429. New York: Wiley.

McRae, D. L., C. L. Branch, B. Milner (1968). The occipital horns and cerebral dominance. *Neurology* 18:95–98.

Mandell, A. J., and S. Knapp (1979). Asymmetry and mood, emergent properties of serotonin regulation. *Arch Gen Psychiat* 36:909–916.

Manz, H. J., T. M. Phillips, G. Rowden, et al. (1979). Unilateral megalencephaly, cerebral cortical dysplasia, neuronal hypertrophy, and heterotopia: Cytomorphometric, fluorometric cytochemical, and biochemical analysis. *Acta Neuropathol* 45:97–103.

Marín-Padilla, M. (1970). Prenatal and early postnatal ontogenesis of the human motor cortex: A Golgi study. I: The sequential development of the cortical layers. *Brain Res* 23:167–183.

Marsh, D. G., D. A. Meyers, and W. B. Bias (1981). The epidemiology and genetics of atopic allergy. *NEJM* 305:1551–1559.

Masala, C., M. A. Amendolea, and R. Lopes (1981). Subclinical hypothyroidism. *Lancet* 1:161.

Masland, R. L., and M. W. Masland (1981). Epilepsy and specific learning disability. *Abstracts, World Congress of Neurology,* Kyoto, 116. Int. Congress Series 548. Amsterdam: Excerpta Medica.

Maugh, T. H., II (1982). A new marker for diabetes. *Science* 215:651.

Maxon, S. C., B. E. Ginsburg, and A. Trattner (1979). Interaction of Y chromosomal and autosomal gene(s) in the development of intermale aggression in mice. *Behav Genet* 9:219–226.

Meisel, R. L., and I. L. Ward (1981). Fetal female rats are masculinized by male littermates located caudally in the uterus. *Science* 213:239–241.

Mellon, DeF. (1981). Nerves and the transformation of claw type in snapping shrimps. *TINS* 4:245–248.

Mendlewicz, J. (1983). Rôle des facteurs neurobiologiques dans le diagnostic et le traitement des syndromes dépressifs. *Bull Mém Acad royal Méd Belgique* 138:169–178.

Mesulam, M.-M. (1981). A cortical network for directed attention and unilateral neglect. *Ann Neurol* 10:309–325.

Mesulam, M.-M. (1982). Slowly progressive aphasia without generalized dementia. *Ann Neurol* 11:592–598.

Meyer, A. (1950). *The Collected Papers of Adolph Meyer*. Baltimore, Md.: The Johns Hopkins Press.

Meyer-Bahlburg, H. F. L., and A. A. Ehrhardt (1980). Sex hormone administration during pregnancy: Behavioral sequelae in the offspring. In *Psychosomatic Obstetrics and Gynaecology*, D. D. Youngs and A. A. Ehrhardt, eds. New York: Appleton-Century-Crofts.

Michaelson, J. (1981). Genetic polymorphism of B2-microglobulin (B2m) maps to the H-3 region of chromosome 2. *Immunogenetics* 13:167–171.

Michaelson, J., A. Ferreira, and V. Nussenzweig (1981). *cis*-Interacting genes of the S region of the murine major histocompatibility complex. *Nature* 289:306–308.

Mieses-Reif, M. (1936). Contents of pigment in hair and iris in its relation to refraction. *Folia Ophthalmol Orientalia* 2:258–260.

Miller, E. (1971). Handedness and the pattern of human ability. *Br J Psychol* 62:111–112.

Milner, B. (1973). Hemispheric specialization: Scope and limits. In *The Neurosciences: Third Study Program*, F. O. Schmitt and F. G. Worden, eds., 75–89. Cambridge, Mass.: The MIT Press.

Minot, G. (1948). Pernicious anemia. In *Textbook of Medicine*, R. L. Cecil, ed., 1091–1098. Philadelphia: W. B. Saunders Co.

Mittwoch, V. (1975). Lateral asymmetry and gonadal differentiation. *Lancet* 1:401–402.

Mohr, J. P., W. C. Watters, and G. W. Duncan (1975). Thalamic hemorrhage and aphasia. *Brain Lang* 2:3–17.

Money, J., and A. A. Ehrhardt (1972). Gender dimorphic behavior and fetal sex hormones. In *Recent Progress in Hormone Research*, vol. 28, E. B. Astwood, ed., 735–754. New York: Academic Press.

Mori, K., H. Handa, H. Gi, et al. (1980). Cavernomas in the middle fossa. *Surg Neurol* 14:21–31.

Mori, K., T. Murata, N. Hashimoto, et al. (1980). Clinical analysis of arteriovenous malformations in children. *Child's Brain* 6:13–25.

Moscovitch, M., and L. C. Smith (1979). Differences in neuronal organization between individuals with inverted and non-inverted handwriting postures. *Science* 205:710–713.

Murgita, R. A., and T. B. Tomasi (1975). Suppression of immune response by alphafetoprotein. *J Exper Med* 141:440–452.

Myers, R. H., D. Goldman, E. D. Bird, et al. (1983). Maternal transmission in Huntington's disease. *Lancet* 1:208–210.

Naeser, M., M. A. Alexander, N. Helm-Estabrooks, et al. (1982). Aphasia with predominantly subcortical lesion sites. *Arch Neurol* 39:2–14.

Naftolin, F. (1981). Understanding the bases of sex differences. *Science* 211:1263–1264.

Nance, W. E. (1969). Anencephaly and spina bifida: A possible example of cytoplasmic inheritance in man. *Nature* 224:373–375.

Narang, H. K. (1977). Right-left asymmetry in myelin development in epiretinal portion of the rabbit optic nerve. *Nature* 266:28–29.

Nasrallah, H. A., K. Keelor, and M. McCalley-Whitters (1983). Laterality shift in alcoholic males. *Biol Psychiatry* 18:1065–1067.

Netley, C. (1977). Dichotic listening of callosal agenesis and Turner's syndrome patients. In *Language Development and Neurological Theory*, S. J. Segalowitz and F. A. Gruber, eds., 133–143. New York: Academic Press.

Netley, C., and J. Rovet (1982). Handedness in 47, XXY males. *Lancet* 2:267.

Neville, A. C. (1976). *Animal Asymmetry*. London: Edward Arnold.

Newlin, D. B., B. Carpenter, and C. J. Golden (1981). Hemispheric asymmetries in schizophrenia. *Biol Psychiatry* 16:561–582.

Newson-Davis, J., and A. Vincent (1982). Receptors, antibodies and disease. *Imm Today* 3:149–152.

Nichols, P. L., and T.-C. Chen (1981). *Minimal Brain Dysfunction: A Prospective Study*. Hillsdale, N.J.: Lawrence Erlbaum.

Nieuwenhuys, R. (1977). The brain of the lamprey in a comparative perspective. In *Evolution and Lateralization of the Brain*, S. J. Dimond and D. A. Blizard, eds., 97–145. New York Academy of Sciences.

Nikkuni, S., Y. Yashima, K. Kishige, et al. (1981). Left-right hemispheric asymmetry of cortical speech zones in the Japanese brain. *Brain Nerve* 33:77–84.

Nora, J. J., A. H. Nora, A. G. Perinchief, et al. (1976). Congenital abnormalities and first-trimester exposure to progestagen/oestrogen. *Lancet* 1:313–314.

Nordeen, E. J., and P. Yahr (1982). Hemispheric asymmetries in the behavioral and hormonal effects of sexually differentiating mammalian brain. *Science* 218:391–393.

Nordeen, E. J., and P. Yahr (1983). A regional analysis of estrogen binding to hypothalamic cell nuclei in relation to masculinization and defeminization. *J Neurosci* 3:933–941.

Nottebohm, F. (1980). Brain pathways for vocal learning in birds: A review of the first 10 years. *Prog Psychobiol Physiol Psychol* 9:85–124.

Nottebohm, F. (1981). A brain for all seasons: Cyclical anatomical changes in song control nuclei of the canary brain. *Science* 214:1368–1370.

Nottebohm, F., and A. P. Arnold (1976). Sexual dimorphism in vocal control areas of the songbird brain. *Science* 194:211–213.

Nottebohm, F., and M. Nottebohm (1976). Left hypoglossal dominance in the control of canary and white-crowned sparrow song. *J Comp Physiol* Ser. A, 108:171–192.

Nussenzweig, R. S. (1982). Parasitic disease as a cause of immunosuppression. *NEJM* 306:423–424.

Nylander, P. P. S. (1978). Causes of high twinning frequencies in Nigeria. In *Twin Research: Biology and Epidemiology*, W. E. Nance, ed., 35–43. New York: A. R. Liss.

Ohno, S. (1977). The original function of MHC antigens as the general plasma membrane anchorage site of organogenesis-directing proteins. *Immunological Rev* 33:59–69.

Ojemann, G. A., and A. A. Ward (1971). Speech representation in ventrolateral thalamus. *Brain* 94:669–680.

Oke, A., R. Keller, I. Mefford, et al. (1978). Lateralization of norepinephrine in human thalamus. *Science* 200:1411–1413.

Oldfield, R. C. (1969). Handedness in musicians. *Br J Psychol* 60:91–99.

Oldfield, R. C. (1971). The assessment and analysis of handedness: The Edinburgh Inventory. *Neuropsychologia* 9:97–113.

Orton, S. T. (1925). "Word-blindness" in school children. *Arch Neurol Psychiat* 14:581–615.

Oswald, I. (1969). Sleep and its disorders. In *Handbook of Clinical Neurology.* Vol. 3: *Disorders of Higher Nervous Activity*, P. J. Vinken and G. W. Bruyn, eds., 80–111. Amsterdam: North-Holland.

Pande, B. S., and I. Singh (1971). One-sided dominance in the upper limbs of human fetuses as evidenced by asymmetry in muscle and bone weight. *J Anat* 109:457–459.

Paolozzi, C. (1970). Hemisphere dominance and asymmetry related to vulnerability of cerebral hemisphere. *Psychiat Digest* 31:61.

Paolozzi, C., and F. Bravaccio (1969). Ripartizione tra i due emisferi olelle anormalità elletroencefalografiche focalizzate. *Acta Neurol* 24:13–28.

Parisi, P., M. Gatti, G. Prinzi, et al. (1983). Familial incidence of twinning. *Nature* 304:626–628.

Parker, G., and S. Walter (1981). Seasonal variation in depressive disorders and suicidal death in New South Wales. *Br J Psychiatry* 140:626–632.

Paul, K. S., E. Hayward, D. M. Barnes, et al. (1984). Progesterone receptors in meningiomas. *J Neurol Neurosurg Psychiatry* 47:103–104.

Penfield, W., and L. Roberts (1959). *Speech and Brain Mechanisms*. Princeton, N.J.: Princeton University Press.

Petersen, M. R., M. D. Beecher, S. R. Zoloth, et al. (1978). Neural lateralization of species-specific vocalizations by Japanese macaques (*Macaca fuscata*). *Science* 202:324–327.

Peterson, J. M. (1979). Left-handedness: Differences between student artists and scientists. *Percept Mot Skills* 48:961–962.

Peterson, J. M., and L. M. Lansky (1974). Left-handedness among architects: Some facts and speculation. *Percept Mot Skills* 38:547–550.

Peterson, J. M., and L. M. Lansky (1980). Success in architecture: Handedness and/or visual thinking. *Percept Mot Skills* 50:1139–1143.

Pfaff, D. W. (1966). Morphological changes in the brains of adult male rats after neonatal castration. *J Endocrin* 36:415–416.

Pfeifer, R. A. (1936). Pathologie der Hörstrahlung und der corticaler Hörsphäre. In *Handbuch de Neurologie*, vol. 6, O. Bumke and O. Forster, eds., 534–626. Berlin: Springer-Verlag.

Pickering, N. J., J. I. Brody, and M. J. Barrett (1981). Von Willebrand syndromes and mitral-valve prolapse. *NEJM* 305:131–134.

Pirozzolo, F. J., and E. C. Hansch (1982). The neurobiology of developmental reading disorders. In *Neurolinguistic Aspects of Reading Disorders*, R. N. Malatesha and P. C. Aaron, eds., 215–232. New York: Academic Press.

Pohl, H. (1965). Temperature regulation and cold acclimation in the golden hamster. *J Appl Physiol* 20:405–410.

Policansky, D. (1982). Flatfishes and the inheritance of asymmetries. *Behav Brain Sci* 5:262–266.

Ponseti, I. V., V. Pedrimi, R. Wynne-Davies, et al. (1976). Pathogenesis of scoliosis. *Clin Ortho* 120:268–280.

Porac, C., and S. Coren (1981). *Lateral Preferences and Human Behavior*. New York: Springer-Verlag.

Poskanser, D. C. (1975). Hemiatrophies and hemihypertrophies. In *Handbook of Clinical Neurology*. Vol. 22: *System Disorders and Atrophies*, P. J. Vinken, G. W. Bruyn, J. M. B. V. Dejong, and H. L. Klawans, eds., 545–554. Amsterdam: North-Holland.

Provins, K. A., A. D. Milner, and P. Kerr (1982). Asymmetry of mammal preference and performance. *Percept Mot Skills* 54:179–194.

Quinan, C. (1921). Sinistrality in relation to high blood pressure and defects of speech. *Arch Int Med* 27:255–261.

Quinan, C. (1922). A study of sinistrality and muscle coordination in musicians, iron workers and others. *Arch Neurol Psychiat* 7:352–360.

Raisman, G., and P. M. Field (1971). Sexual dimorphism in the preoptic area of the rat. *Science* 173:731–733.

Raisman, G., and P. M. Field (1973). Sexual dimorphism in the neuropil of the preoptic area of the rat and its dependence on neonatal androgen. *Brain Res* 54:1–29.

Rasmussen, T., and B. Milner (1977). The role of early left-brain injury in determining lateralization of cerebral speech functions. In *Evolution and Lateralization of the Brain*, S. J. Dimond and D. A. Blizard, eds., 355–369. New York Academy of Sciences.

Ratcliff, G., C. Dila, L. Taylor, et al. (1980). The morphological asymmetry of the hemispheres and cerebral dominance for speech: A possible relationship. *Brain Lang* 11:87–98.

Rebeiz, J. J., E. H. Kolodny, and E. P. Richardson (1968). Corticodentatonigral degeneration with neuronal achromasia. *Arch Neurol* 18:20–33.

Regli, F., G. Filippa, and M. Wiesendanger (1967). Hereditary mirror movements. *Arch Neurol* 16:620–623.

Reiter, R. J. (1980). The pineal gland and its hormones in the control of reproduction in mammals. *Endocrine Reviews* 1:109–131.

Renoux, G., K. Bizière, M. Renoux, et al. (1983a). The production of T-Cell-Inducing factors in mice is controlled by brain neocortex. *Scand J Immunol* 17:45–50.

Renoux, G., K. Bizière, M. Renoux, et al. (1983b). A balanced brain symmetry modulates T cell-mediated events. *J Neuroimmunol* 5:227–238.

Rey, P. (1885). Du poids des lobes cérébraux (frontaux, occipitaux et pariéto-temporaux) d'après le registre de Broca. *Rev d'Anthropol* 8:385–396.

Rich, A. (1982). Right-handed and left-handed DNA: Conformational information in genetic material. *Cold Spring Harbor Symposium on Quantitative Biology* 47:1–12.

Rimland, B. (1964). *Infantile Autism*. New York: Appleton-Century-Crofts.

Rimland, B. (1978). The autistic savant. *Psychol Today* (Aug), 69–80.

Robinson, T. E., J. B. Becker, D. M. Camp, et al. (1985). Variation in the pattern of behavioral and brain asymmetries due to sex differences. In Glick, ed. (1985), 185–231.

Robinson, T. E., J. B. Becker, and V. D. Ramirez (1980). Sex differences in amphetamine-elicited rotational behavior and lateralization of striatal dopamine in rats. *Brain Res Bull* 5:539–545.

Rodbard, D. (1981). The role of regional body temperature in the pathogenesis of disease. *NEJM* 305:808–814.

Rogers, L. J. (1980). Lateralization in the avian brain. *Bird Behav* 2:1–12.

Rogers, L. J. (1982). Light experience and asymmetry of brain function in chickens. *Nature* 297:223–225.

Rosen, G. D., A. S. Berrebi, D. A. Yutzey, et al. (1983). Prenatal testosterone causes shift of asymmetry in neonatal tail posture of the rat. *Devel Brain Res* 9:99–101.

Rosenberg, C. A., G. H. Derman, W. C. Grabb, et al. (1983). Hypomastia and mitral-valve prolapse. *NEJM* 309:1230–1232.

Rosenberger, P. B., and D. B. Hier (1980). Cerebral asymmetry and verbal intellectual deficits. *Ann Neurol* 8:300–304.

Rosman, N. P., and B. A. Kakulas (1966). Mental deficiency associated with muscular dystrophy. *Brain* 89:769–788.

Ross, M. H., A. M. Galaburda, and T. L. Kemper (1984). Down's syndrome: Is there a decreased population of neurons? *Neurology* 34:909–916.

Rubens, A. B., M. W. Mahowald, and J. T. Hutton (1976). Asymmetry of the lateral sylvian fissures in man. *Neurology* 26:620–624.

Sai-Halasz, A., G. Brunecker, and S. T. Szara (1958). Dymethyltryptamin: Ein neues Psychoticum. *Psychiatr Neurol (Basel)* 135:285–301.

Samarel, A., T. L. Wright, F. Sergay, et al. (1976). Thalamic hemorrhage with speech disorder. *Trans Am Neurol Assoc* 101:283–285.

Sano, F. (1918). James Henry Pullen, The Genius of Earlswood. *J Mental Sci* 64:251–267.

Satz, P. (1973). Left-handedness and early brain insult: An explanation. *Neuropsychologia* 2:115–117.

Satz, P. (1980). Incidence of aphasia in lefthanders: A test of some hypothetical models of cerebral speech organization. In *Neuropsychology of Lefthandedness*, J. Herron, ed., 189–198. New York: Academic Press.

Satz, P., Achenbach, and E. Fennel (1967). Correlations between assessed manual laterality and predicted speech laterality in a normal population. *Neuropsychologia* 5:295–310.

Saxen, L., and S. Toivonen (1962). *Primary Embryonic Induction*. London: Logos.

Schachter, S. C., and A. M. Galaburda (in press). Development and biological associations of cerebral dominance: Review and possible mechanisms. *J Amer Acad Child Psychiat.*

Schaeffer, A. A. (1928). Spiral movement in man. *J Morph* 45:293–398.

Scheibel, A. M. (1984). A dendritic correlate of human speech. In Geschwind and Galaburda, eds. (1984), 43–52.

Schnall, B. S., and D. W. Smith (1974). Nonrandom laterality of malformations in paired structures. *J Ped* 83:509–511.

Schneider, G. E. (1981). Early lesions and abnormal neuronal connections: Developmental rules can lead axons astray, with functional consequences. *TINS* 4:187–192.

Schneider, L. H., R. B. Murphy, and E. E. Coons (1982). Lateralization of striatal dopamine (D2) receptors in normal rats. *Neurosci Lett* 33:281–284.

Schoene, W. C., S. Carpenter, P. O. Behan, et al. (1977). "Onion-bulb" formations in the central and peripheral nervous system in association with multiple sclerosis and hypertrophic polyneuropathy. *Brain* 100:755–773.

Scott, W. J., R. E. Butcher, C. W. Kindt, et al. (1972). Greater sensitivity of female than male rat embryos to acetazolamide teratogenicity. *Teratology* 6:239–240.

Sedgwick, R. P., and E. Boder (1972). Ataxia-telangiectasia. In *Handbook of Clinical Neurology.* Vol. 14: *The Phakomatoses,* P. J. Vinken and G. W. Bruyn, eds., 267–339. Amsterdam: North-Holland.

Seltzer, B., and I. Sherwin (1983). A comparison of clinical features in early- and late-onset primary degenerative dementia. *Arch Neurol* 40:143–146.

Selye, H. (1971). *Hormones and Resistance.* Vols. 1 and 2. New York: Springer-Verlag.

Serafetinides, E. A. (1965). The significance of the temporal lobes and of hemispheric dominance in the production of LSD-25 symptomatology in man. *Neuropsychologia* 3:69–79.

Shapiro, A. K., and E. Shapiro (1982). An update on Tourette syndrome. *Am J Psychotherapy* 36:378–391.

Sherman, G. F., and A. M. Galaburda (1982). Cortical volume asymmetry and behavior in the albino rat. *Soc Neurosci Abstr* 8:627.

Sherman, G. F., and A. M. Galaburda (1984). Neocortical asymmetry and open-field behavior in the rat. *Exp Neurol* 86:473–482.

Sherman, G. F., J. A. Garbanati, G. D. Rosen, et al. (1980). Brain and behavioral asymmetries for spatial preference in rats. *Brain Res* 192:61–67.

Sherwin, I., P. Peron-Magnan, J. Bancaud, et al. (1982). Prevalence of psychosis in epilepsy as a function of the laterality of the epileptogenic lesion. *Arch Neurol* 39:621–625.

Shimizu, A., and M. Endo (1983). Handedness and familial sinistrality in a Japanese student population. *Cortex* 19:265–272.

Simpson, E. (1983). Antigens associated with H-2 embryos and tumours. *Nature* 306:738–739.

Singh, I. (1971). One-sided dominance in the limbs of rabbits and frogs, as evidenced by asymmetry of bone weight. *J Anat* 109:271–275.

Smith, G. E. (1904). A preliminary note on an aberrant circumolivary bundle springing from the left pyramidal tract. *Rev Neurol Psychiat* 2:377–383.

Smith, S. D., W. J. Kimberling, B. F. Pennington, et al. (1983). Specific reading disability: Identification of an inherited form through linkage analysis. *Science* 219:1345–1347.

Sohnle, P. G., and S. R. Gambert (1982). Thermoneutrality: An evolutionary advantage against ageing. *Lancet* 1:1099–1011.

Solomon, F. (1979). Detailed neurite morphologies of sister neuroblastoma cells are related. *Cell* 16:165–169.

Sonnhag, C., E. Karlsson, and J. Hed (1979). Procainamide-induced lupus erythematosus-like syndrome in relation to acetylator phenotype and plasma levels of procainamide. *Acta Med Scand* 206:245–251.

Sperry, R. W. (1950). Neuronal specificity. In *Genetic Neurology*, P. Weiss, ed., 232–239. Chicago: University of Chicago Press.

Starr, M. S., and K. Kilpatrick (1981). Bilateral asymmetry in brain GABA function? *Neurosci Lett* 25:167–172.

Staunton, T., P. Fedio, and P. Kornblith (1985). Developmental history of brain tumors: Evidence of early neurological dysfunction in adults with malignant gliomas. *Ann Neurol* 18:110.

Stefan, M., S. Milea, S. Magureanu, et al. (1981). The autistic syndrome and epileptic seizures, clinical and etiopathogenetic interference. *Rev Med Interna (Neurol Psychiatr)* 26:205–211.

Stejskal, L., and Z. Tomanek (1981). Postural laterality in torticollis and torsion dystonia. *J Neurol Neurosurg Psychiatry* 44:1029–1034.

Stimson, W. H., and P. J. Crilly (1981). Effects of steroids on the secretion of immunoregulatory factors by thymic epithelial cell cultures. *Immunology* 44:401–407.

Stokes, K. A., and D. C. McIntyre (1981). Lateralized asymmetrical state-dependent learning produced by kindled convulsions from the rat hippocampus. *Physiol Behav* 26:163–169.

Strauss, E., and C. Fitz (1980). Occipital horn asymmetry in children. *Ann Neurol* 8:437:439.

Strongin, A. C., and R. W. Guillery (1981). The relationship of melanin distribution to cellular degeneration in the developing mammalian eye. *J Neurosci* 1:1193–1204.

Strub, R., and N. Geschwind (1971). Gerstmann syndrome without aphasia. *Cortex* 10:378–387.

Stumpf, W. E., M. Sar, D. A. Keefer, et al. (1976). The anatomical substrate of neuroendocrine regulation as defined by autoradiography with ^{3}H-estradiol, ^{3}H-testosterone, ^{3}H-dihydrotestosterone and ^{3}H-progesterone. In *Neuroendocrine Regulation of Fertility* (International Symposium, Simla, 1974). Basel: Karger.

Suzuki, J., and S. Komatsu (1981). New embolization method using estrogen for dural arteriovenous malformation and meningioma. *Neurology* 16:438–442.

Swinson, C. M., G. Slavin, E. C. Coles, et al. (1983). Coeliac disease and malignancy. *Lancet* 1:111–115.

Szara, S. (1957). The comparison of the psychotic effect of tryptamine derivates with the effects of mescaline and LSD-25 in self experiments. In *Psychotropic Drugs*, S. A. Garattini and V. Ghetti, eds., 460. Amsterdam: Elsevier.

Szondi, L. (1932). Konstitutionsanalyse von 100 Stotterern. *Wien med Wchnschr* 82:922–928.

Takei, Y., M. Kurisaka, G. S. Pearl, et al. (1981). Estrogen receptors in malignant gliomas. *Proc World Congress of Neurology*, Kyoto.

Talal, N. (1977a). Immunologic and viral factors in autoimmune diseases. *Medical Clinics of North America* 61:205–215.

Talal, N. (1977b). *Autoimmunity*. New York: Academic Press.

Taylor, D. C. (1969). Differential rates of cerebral maturation between sexes and between hemispheres. *Lancet* 2:140–142.

Taylor, D. C. (1974). The influence of sexual differentiation on growth, development, and disease. In *Scientific Foundations of Paediatrics*, J. A. Davis and J. Dobbing, eds., 29–44. Philadelphia: W. B. Saunders Co.

Taylor, D. C. (1975a). Factors influencing the occurrence of schizophrenia-like psychosis in patients with temporal lobe epilepsy. *Psychol Med* 5:249–254.

Taylor, D. C. (1975b). Ontogenesis of chronic epileptic psychoses: A reanalysis. *Psychol Med* 1:247–253.

Taylor, D. C. (1976). Developmental stratagems organising intellectual skills: Evidence from studies of temporal lobectomy for epilepsy. In *The Neuropsychology of Learning Disorders*, R. M. Knights and D. Bakker, eds., 149–171. University Park, Md.: University Park Press.

Taylor, D. C. (1981). Brain lesions, surgery, seizures and mental symptoms. In *Psychiatry of Epilepsy*, E. Reynolds and M. Trimble, eds. Edinburgh: Churchill Livingstone.

Taylor, D. C., and W. P. Faulk (1981). Prevention of recurrent abortions with leucocyte transfusions. *Lancet* 2:68–69.

Taylor, D. C., and C. Ounsted (1971). Biological mechanisms influencing the outcome of seizures in response to fever. *Epilepsia* 12:33–45.

Taylor, R. A. (1960). Heredofamilial mononeuritis multiplex with brachial predilection. *Brain* 83:113–137.

Teng, E. L., P.-H. Lee, and K.-S. Yang (1976). Handedness in a Chinese population. *Science* 193:1148–1150.

Teszner, D., A. Tzavaras, J. Gruner, et al; (1972). L'asymétrie droite gauche du planum temporale: À propos de l'étude anatomique de 100 cerveaux. *Rev Neurol* (Paris) 146:444–449.

Theofilopoulos, A. G., G. J. Prud'Homme, T. M. Fieser, et al. (1983). B-cell hyperactivity in murine lupus. I. Immunological abnormalities in lupus-prone strains and the activation of normal B-cells. *Imm Today* 4:287–291.

Thonnard-Neumann, E. (1969). Some interrelationships of vasoactive substances and basophilic leukocytes in migraine headache. *Headache* 9:130–140.

Tieche, M., G. A. Lupi, F. Gutzwiller, et al. (1981). Borderline low thyroid function and thyroid autoimmunity. *Br Heart J* 46:202–206.

Tisserand, (1944) Dominance latérale et bec-de-lièvre. *Arch françaises Pédiatrie* II: 166–167.

Tisserand, M. (1949). Résultats d'études statistiques sur les becs-de-lièvre. *Semaine des hôpitaux de Paris* 25:2547–2550.

Tissot, R., J. Constantinidis, and J. Richard (1975). *La maladie de Pick*. Paris: Masson et Cie.

Toone, B. K., M. Wheeler, M. Nanjee, et al. (1983). Sex hormones, sexual activity and plasma convulsant levels in male epileptics. *J Neurol Neurosurg Psychiatry* 46:824–826.

Toran-Allerand, C. D. (1978). Gonadal hormones and brain development: Cellular aspects of sexual differentiation. *Amer Zool* 18:553–565.

Torch, W. C., A. Hirano, and S. Solomon (1977). Anterograde transneuronal degeneration in the limbic system: Clinical-anatomic correlation. *Neurology* 27:1157–1163.

Trentham, D. E. (1976). Letter: Berry aneurysm and lupus. *NEJM* 295:114.

Tryphonas, H., and R. Trites (1979). Food allergy in children with hyperactivity, learning disabilities and/or minimal brain dysfunction. *Ann Allergy* 42:22–27.

Tucker, H. A., and R. K. Ringer (1982). Controlled photoperiodic environments for food animals. *Science* 216:1381–1386.

Valdes, J. J., C. Mactatus, R. N. Cory, et al. (1981). Lateralization of norepinephrine, serotonin, and choline uptake into hippocampal synaptosomes of sinistral rats. Physiol Behav 27:381–383.

Vandenberg, S. G., and A. R. Kuse (1979). Spatial ability: A critical review of the sex-linked major gene hypothesis. In *Sex-Related Differences in Cognitive Functioning*, M. A. Wittig and A. C. Petersen, eds., 67–94. New York: Academic Press.

Veith, G., and W. Schwindt (1976). Pathologisch-anatomischer Beitrag zum Problem "Nichtsesshaftigkeit." *Fortschritte Neurol-Psychiat* 44:1–21.

Verkoren, A. C. (1983). Oorsprang van links-en rechtshandigheid wordt duidelijker. *Aarde & Kosmos* 2:158–160.

Vetter, V. L., and W. J. Raskind (1983). Congenital complete heart block and connective tissue disease. *NEJM* 309:236–237.

Vrensen, G., and D. deGroot (1974). The effects of dark rearing and its recovery on synaptic terminals in the visual cortex of rabbits. A quantitative electron microscopic study. *Brain Res* 78:263–278.

Waber, D. P. (1976). Sex differences in cognition: A function of maturation rate? *Science* 192:572–574.

Waber, D. P. (1981). Environmental influences on brain and behavior. In *Sex Differences in Dyslexia*, A. Ansara, et al., eds., 73–79. Towsen, Md.: The Orton Dyslexia Society.

Wada, J. A., R. Clarke, and A. Hamm (1975). Cerebral hemispheric asymmetry in humans. *Arch Neurol* 32:239–246.

Wada, J. A., and A. E. Davies (1977). Fundamental nature of human infant's brain asymmetry. *Can J Neurol Sci* 4:203–207.

Wada, J. A., and T. Rasmussen (1960). Intracarotid injection of sodium amytal for the lateralization of cerebral speech dominance. *J Neurosurg* 17:266–282.

Wahlsten, D. (1981). Mice in utero while mother is lactating suffer higher frequency of defective corpus callosum. *Neurosci Abstr* 7:349.

Walter, C. W., and V. J. Dovey (1947). Clinical and EEG studies of temporal lobe function. *Proc Roy Soc Med* 42:891–904.

Ward, I. L., and J. Weisz (1980). Maternal stress alters plasma testosterone in fetal males. *Science* 207:328–329.

Warner, N. L., A. Szenberg, and F. M. Burnet (1962). The immunological role of different lymphoid organs in the chicken. *Austral J Exp Biol Med Sci* 40:373–388.

Wasi, P., and M. Block (1961). The histopathological study of the development of the irradiation-induced leukemia in C57BL mice and of its inhibition by testosterone. *Cancer Res* 21:463–473.

Waxman, S. G., and N. Geschwind (1975). The interictal behavior syndrome of temporal lobe epilepsy. *Arch Gen Psychiat* 32:1580–1586.

Waziri, R. (1980). Lateralization of neuroleptic-induced dyskinesia indicates pharmacological asymmetry in the brain. *Psychopharmacology* 68:51–53.

Weber, W. W., and D. W. Hein (1979). Clinical pharmacokinesis of isoniazid. *Clin Pharmokinetics* 4:401–422.

Webster, W. G., and I. H. Webster (1975). Anatomical asymmetry of the cerebral hemispheres of the cat brain. *Physiol Behav* 14:867–869.

Weinberger, D. R., D. J. Luchins, J. Morihisa, et al. (1982). Asymmetrical volume of the right and left frontal and occipital regions of the human brain. *Ann Neurol* 11:97–100.

Weintraub, S., and M.-M. Mesulam (1983). Developmental learning disabilities of the right hemisphere. *Arch Neurol* 40:463–468.

Weston, J. A. (1970). The migration and differentiation of neural crest cells. *Advances Morph* 8:41–114.

Willis, R. A. (1960). *The Pathology of the Tumours of Children*. London: Oliver and Boyd.

Witelson, S. F., and W. Pallie (1973). Left hemisphere specialization for language in the newborn: Neuroanatomical evidence of asymmetry. *Brain* 96:641–646.

Witkop, C. J., Jr., B. Jay, D. Crul, et al. (1982). Optic neurological abnormalities in oculocutaneous and ocular albinism. *Birth Defects* 18:299–316.

Wittig, M. A., and A. C. Petersen, eds. (1979). *Sex-related Differences in Cognitive Function*. New York: Academic Press.

Woo, T. L. (1931). On the asymmetry of the human skull. *Biometrika* 22:324–352.

Wood, L. C. (1983). Presentation, American Thyroid Association, New Orleans.

Woods, B. T., and M. D. Eby (1982). Excessive mirror movements and aggression. *Biol Psychiatry* 17:23–32.

Woods, B. T., and H.-L. Teuber (1978). Mirror movements after childhood hemiparesis. *Neurology* 28:1152–1157.

Wynne-Davies, R. (1978). Heritable disorders in orthopedics. *Orth Clin North America* 9:3–9.

Yakovlev, P. I., and P. Rakic (1966). Patterns of decussation of bulbar pyramids and distribution of pyramidal tracts on two sides of the spinal cord. *Trans Am Neurol Assoc* 91:366–367.

Yeni-Komshian, G. H., and D. A. Benson (1976). Anatomical study of cerebral asymmetry in the temporal lobe of humans, chimpanzees, and rhesus monkeys. *Science* 192:387–389.

Zangwill, O. (1960). *Cerebral Dominance and Its Relation to Psychological Function.* Springfield, Ill.: Charles C. Thomas.

Zimmerberg, B., A. J. Strumpf, and S. D. Glick (1978). Cerebral asymmetry and left-right discrimination. *Brain Res* 140:194–196.

Zimmerberg, B., S. D. Glick, and T. P. Jerussi (1974). Neurochemical correlate of a spatial preference in rats. *Science* 185:623–625.

Index

Acquired immune deficiency syndrome (AIDS), 175–176
Afzelius, B.A., 233, 235
Agranoff, B.W., 231
Alcoholism, 210
Alexander, M.A., 160
Alien tissue. *See* Congenital anomalies; Tissue factors
Allergies. *See* Atopic disorders
Alopecia areata, 194
Alphafetoprotein, 110, 119–120, 172. *See also* Sex hormones
Altschule, M.D., 221
Alzheimer's disease, 192, 207–208
Amaducci, L.S., 39, 41, 215
Ames, L.B., 78
Amphetamines, 211, 213
ANA test, 195–196
Anatomical asymmetry. *See also* specific brain structures
  as basic, 127–129
  degrees of, 33
  and fetal development, 10–11, 40–43, 46–47
  in humans, 21–35
  independence in, 32–33
  in nonhuman species, 3, 7, 48–53
Anchoring sites, 121
Aneurysms, and immune system, 187
Angiomas, spinal cord, 187
Animal models. *See* Nonhuman species
Annett, M., 3, 6, 14, 68–71, 74–75, 79, 126–128, 133, 138, 235–236
Annual cycles, 218–221
Anomalous dominance. *See also* Random dominance
  assessment of, 74
  defined, 67–72
  and ethnic differences, 144–146
  and lefthandedness, 70
  and motor dominance, 78–79
  and self-described handedness, 72–73

Anorexia nervosa, 86
Antigens, and immune attack, 119–121, 185–186, 193–197, 208. *See also* H-Y antigen; Immune response
Antinuclear antibody (ANA) test, 195–196
Aphasia, 5–6, 33, 192, 207–208
Arachnoid cysts, 187–188
Architectonic areas, 35–38. *See also* Area Tpt
Area Tpt (temporoparietal)
  and pharmacological asymmetry, 39, 214
  size asymmetry of, 2, 37, 214
  and Wernicke's area, 36
Arteriovenous malformation (AVM), 62
Artistic ability, lack of, 87
Asymmetry
  advantages of, 20–21
  independence in, 238
  linked, 225, 227, 237–239
  in molecular physics, 225–227, 230–231
  reverse, 236
  in single cells, 227–230, 234
Ataxia telangiectasia, 120, 174
Atopic disorders, 4, 13, 88, 91–92. *See also* Immune disorders
Attentional systems, 45
Autism, 83, 85–86. *See also* Learning disorders
Autoimmune disorders, 13, 88, 118, 122–123. *See also* Immune disorders
Autonomic activities, 45
AVM. *See* Arteriovenous malformation
Axial dominance, 77–79

Baboon, 49, 50, 205–206
Badian, N.A., 117, 135, 219
Bakan, P., 72, 210
Balthasar, K., 65
Beaussart, M., 205
Beck, E., 213

Bradford Books

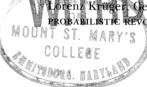